SCARS

AN ANTHOLOGY

"Scars offers an eclectic range of deeply personal meditations on pain, skin, and often but not always, healing. Each voice seeks to make sense of visible, tactile memories of pain, claiming scars as essential to the person they have become. Collectively, these voices give testimony to the connection between self-expression and resilience."

—Arthur W. Frank, *The Wounded Storyteller: Body, Illness, and Ethics,* and *At the Will of the Body: Reflections on Illness*

———✝———

"If scars are the memory of pain, then this volume is a body of those memories recollected as stories—stories as compelling, as vivid, as dramatic as the thing, the scar, itself."

—Lisa Sanders, Yale School of Medicine, the doctor behind *House, M.D.* and *New York Times* "Diagnosis" Columnist, author of *Every Patient Tells a Story: Medical Mysteries and the Art of Diagnosis*

———✝———

"The stories here are, as you would imagine of a book on scars, brave, painful, cathartic, and intense—intensely moving. We see the ways lives fall apart, they ways they are stitched back together, and the scars left by those fractured and transformative moments. Read these stories with caution, pace yourself: they are hard stories, difficult stories. After a session of reading you will feel that your own skin has been cut open, post-accident or post-diagnosis or otherwise. But they are important stories, necessary stories; the kind of stories that make us less alone in our own skin, less alone in our moments of fear and trauma and loss."

—Arianne Zwartjes, *Detailing Trauma: A Poetic Anatomy, The Surfacing of Excess, disem(body): a tracing,* and *(Stitched) A Surface Opens*

———/———

"Scars digs deep, and from many directions, into what it means to hurt, to heal, to keep on going. I came away from this anthology feeling that it had opened up a new space in which to confront our relationship with our bodies, with imperfection, with vulnerability and fragility and strength. This is an expansive book, and a necessary one."
—Yael Goldstein Love, *The Passion of Tasha Darsky*

———/———

'Scars ground us to our pasts and our bodies like little else. Wood has expertly cultivated a rich collection of powerful and touching stories from a diversity of voices. You won't look at your own skin the same way again."
—Matthew Hutson, *The 7 Laws of Magical Thinking: How Irrational Beliefs Keep Us Happy, Healthy, and Sane*

———/———

SCARS

AN ANTHOLOGY

Edited by
Erin Wood

May you scars shine

et alia press

Little Rock, Arkansas

2015

Published in the United States of America by:
Et Alia Press
1819 Shadow Lane
Little Rock, AR 72207

etaliapress.com

ISBN: 978-0-9828184-7-3
Library of Congress Control Number: 2015945487

Cover Image by: David Jay
Cover Design by: Jesse Nickles
Scarbill Design by: Kathy Oliverio

PERMISSIONS AND ACKNOWLEDGEMENTS

Marcus Cafagña: "Something Faithful," originally published in *The Broken World* (1996), reprinted with permission of the author and University of Illinois Press.

Jill Christman: "Burned Images," originally published in *Darkroom: A Family Exposure* (2002), reprinted with permission of the author and University of Georgia Press.

Chelsey Clammer: "Cut," originally published in another version in *The Rumpus* October 1, 2012, reprinted with permission of the author and *The Rumpus*.

Jesse Nickels: "Portrait of Otto Skorzeny" and "This is the Enemy." Illustrations printed in "My Schmiss" with permission of illustrator.

Jim Ferris: "Scars, A Love Story," full-length solo performance originally performed at Ithaca College, the University of Toledo, the National Communication Association convention in San Francisco, 2010; the University of Toledo, Access Living/Chicago, the Ohio State University, the Society for Disability Studies conference in San Jose, 2011; University of Puerto Rico Rio Piedras, 2012; Association for Higher Education and Disability conference, Baltimore, 2013; substantially abbreviated, revised, and printed with permission of the author.

David Jay: Commentary and images displayed worldwide, reprinted with permission of the photographer.

Peter Mulvey: "The Trouble with Poets." *The Trouble with Poets*, © 2000 by Signature Sounds, B000S5B2CM, compact disc. Partial lyrics printed in "Scars: A Love Story" with permission of songwriter.

Jeffrey Paolano: "The Corpsman," originally published in another version in *O-Dark-Thirty* July 17, 2014, reprinted with permission of the author and *O-Dark-Thirty* <o-dark-thirdy.org>.

Erin Wood: "We Scar, We Heal, We Rise," originally published on anderbo.com, as a finalist for the 2011–2012 Anderbo Creative Nonfiction Prize, reprinted with permission of the author.

TABLE OF CONTENTS

PREFACE

Welcome to *Scars: An Anthology*.

A question that has prodded me again and again throughout the editing of this volume is: *To whom do our scars belong?* My personal answer must have obscured my own singular thinking for all the years leading up to this project: my scars belong to me. They are "my scars." But in collecting scar stories, I have learned this is hardly everyone's truth.

Just as the events surrounding and the stories about scars belong at once to their narrators and to other people and situations within and without narrators' control, there is a great deal about our scars that extends far beyond the individual body and the self. For Heidi Andrea Restrepo Rhodes, the mark at the nape of her neck belongs to her ancestors, reaching to her across generations as an emblem of their "treacherous strides." For Natalie Karneef, the emptiness left on her body from a mole she chose to remove speaks of a reclaiming of her body, her story, her life from her mother, who bore the same mole in the same place. For physician and surgeon Brian Burton, scars created by his hand are labeled "my scars," a reminder that some might claim ownership of the scars on another's body, even that others can learn and know our bodies in ways that we ourselves may not.[1] This notion might even be disturbing—sometimes our bodies have endured traumas our minds do not recall, and yet our bodies serve up those obscured or forgotten interludes in the form of scars. Perhaps an example of this phenomenon, Douglas Kidd grammatically constructs a distanced relationship: "The scars I have," and "the scars I possess," he says about the external and internal marks left on his body following a near-fatal collision and its accompanying brain surgery. Similarly, Michelle Jarvis references "the scars" in speaking of the physical reminders of her colon cancer. Might these ways of talking about the marks of our lives indicate that for some of us, scars are things lived with rather than fully integrated into our being? Something *on* rather than *part of* our bodies? Scars may even belong to different versions of ourselves: our past selves (Chelsey Clammer, Lea Ervin, Kelli Dunham, Jason Wiest), or new selves (Natalie Karneef, Philip Martin), selves in transition (Jim Ferris, Aimee Ross, Jen Stager, Andrea Zekis), or even selves we wish to regard more fully (Lorrie Fredette, Melissa Nicolas). Other relationships with scars may be beyond language; I sent photographer David Jay a list of interview questions but quickly realized I was attempting to foist my perspective upon him: while I understand the world through words, he understands the world through images, and naturally desires that his images speak for themselves in translating and reflecting his mode(s) of understanding. His photographs *are* his interview. Although it is perhaps impossible to edit without bias, I tried my utmost to honor each voice by acknowledging particular and individual relationships with their own scars and the scars of others, as evinced through contributors' own choices of words and approaches indicating these relationships. This volume and these authors have raised the question *To whom do our scars belong?* and so many other lines of inquiry well worth following. All the questions they raise seem to point to one answer: there is no correct way, no one way to understand scars.

The volume opens with "Burned Images," the first chapter from Jill Christman's AWP Award-winning memoir, *Darkroom: A Family Exposure*. I've long admired how this piece so artfully and transparently tracks Christman's attempt to pin down "the truth" of a family story that looms large. It hauntingly reveals the many shortcomings of memory and also draws into parallel the transfixing elements of both scars and stories that will resurface throughout the collection. I elected not to divide the book into labeled sections but tried to relate each piece to the next and, in most cases, to the several that surround it in an attempt to provide a constellation of meaning for readers. The first group situates scars within the context of relationships—familial (Jill Christman, Annie Tucker, Marcus Cafagña, Rianne Pallazollo), filial (Gretchen Case, me), spousal (Lea Ervin, Jen Stager), and academic (Shireen Campell). The next grouping addresses more personal struggles with scars, exploring self-mutilation and recovery (Chelsey Clammer, Kelli Dunham), and emotions about scars that fall along a spectrum from disgust to respect (Michelle Jarvis, Samantha Plakun, Aimee Ross, Douglas Kidd). The third group addresses issues of culture, geography, history, and religion (Lorrie Fredette, Heidi Andrea Restrepo Rhodes, Sayantani DasGupta). David Jay's two collections of images depicting mastectomy scars following breast cancer diagnosis and veterans of the Iraq war are flanked by narratives of breast cancer (LaNita Rippere) and war (Jeffrey Paolano). Bennett Battle's "Where the Bodies are Kept" delves into the specter of the medical school anatomy class tradition of meeting one's cadaver, beginning several physician and veterinary narratives that include ObGyn Brian Burton's interview about operating on an Orangutan (his "hairiest patient"), veterinarian Andrea Razer's marveling at the mystery and magic of healing in the animal kingdom, Clairese Webb's facing her own cancer diagnosis while a med student, and Jackie Conger's experience performing C-sections. Beginning with "At the Women's Table: An Interview with Andrea Zekis," readers will discover scars as part of authors' coming of age stories and as shaping gender roles and expectations (Melissa Nicolas, Emilie Staat, Heidi Kim, Jason Wiest, Maurice Carlos Ruffin, Philip Martin, James S. Baumlin, Chris Osmond, Scott Huler). Steve McNamee's review of *Violet*, the musical, is followed by the partial script of Jim Ferris's performance piece, "Scars: A Love Story." My own 2012 prose poem, which in many ways helped mobilize my dreams of a scar anthology, ends the collection. Certainly, many of these pieces cross the very general boundaries I've outlined and could naturally fall into other categories, which is why it made sense to me not to explicitly delineate them. It was also a challenge to confine these pieces to a particular order because those that appear toward the end constitute beginnings in the fresh way they ask us to (re)consider those pieces that appear at the beginning. I envision a web of connections between all the contributions that liberates them from their linear presentation.

As I have asked myself periodically throughout the nearly two years I've been assembling this collection "by what warrant"[2] I was doing so, I sometimes had my doubts. At times, that doubt led me to question the ethicality of pushing others to tell (and re-tell through the editing process) their often deeply painful stories.[3] At other times, the question became, "*What qualifies me for this task?*" I have always returned to this: If I have these questions, this burning need to explain what scars mean, others must too. If we are to make sense of our own scarred bodies, our scar stories, and ourselves, we must necessarily take in and grapple with the stories of others. So my warrant is to act on behalf of others, becoming a medium for their stories. My warrant is that I am one of countless scarred people on this planet. Not only have my scars influenced and impacted me in profound and powerful ways, meaning that the assembling of this collection also constitutes a personal voyage of discovery, but I must provide the confluence of voices on scarring if I hope to initiate a more specialized understanding of what scars mean beyond the "our scars make us stronger" trope.

The authors in this volume are diverse in age, ethnicity, socioeconomic background, gender, sexual orientation, nationality, and occupation. They are also diverse in writing experience; while many are award-winning, prolific professional writers, this represents the first publication for some.

Others are between those poles. It was important to me to offer equal footing for stories to be told, regardless of publishing experience. While all authors currently reside in the United States or Canada, many were born in, often travel to, or are strongly influenced by countries around the globe. Some writings were solicited from authors known and unknown to me, while others found the anthology through calls for submissions on listservs and social media, or even by word of mouth from friends and family. Of note, all entries were gathered on a zero advertising budget. In this way, *Scars* became (as many anthologies must) a community project, with additional investments by many beyond its pages. In organic and informative ways, it also includes the countless stories I have gathered through conversation that were not ultimately printed herein.

I express deepest gratitude for the authors, who have generously given of their time and energies to contribute to this volume because of their genuine belief in the necessity of its creation. I am humbled that my hesitant question, "*Would you consider including your scar story?*" electronically communicated to strangers, has resulted not only in enthusiastic responses and submissions, but in the formation of friendships and alliances. Through the editing process, I have come to know so many authors in intimate and unexpected ways, and I pay homage to all that they have offered up of their words and themselves. I intend for readers to hear these authors voices individually, but also to consider how each selection advances a broader understanding of what scars mean in people's lives and as part of our embodied human experience.

I wish to acknowledge Gretchen Case, Sayantani DasGupta, and Lorrie Fredette, especially, for trusting me enough to jump aboard at the very beginning of this project. Your incredible work led others to join. I also owe a great deal to those authors who finally yielded to my unrelenting pressure to contribute. The encouragement of a most extraordinary teacher, Dr. Toran Isom, invited me to track down sparks of interest to determine where they might lead me; she no doubt served as this book's midwife. Thanks to Jill Christman who indulged a fan without first considering me a stalker, and generously read drafts of "Tissue," sending messages of support and affection from Muncie that I'll always treasure. Thank you to my partners in *Et Alia* Press, George H. Jensen and James S. Baumlin, for supporting me and making numerous important contributions that have made this book possible. A huge hug to Jamie Jensen who says beautiful things that light my way. A nod to Elaine Ruth Boe, who lassoed a great poem and tried with all her wares to track down a plastic surgeon to contribute; perhaps in Volume II! My heels click together as I salute Kathy Oliverio—a rare woman who just plain gets things done. I appreciate all those who in passing or through more extended interactions have encouraged me to follow through. I embrace my husband with deepest affection for enduring my enthusiasm and supporting me in my creative endeavors; his love makes me believe I can pull anything off. I thank my step-father, who is as great a father as a girl could ask for, and who always sees beyond the scars. And perhaps I owe the greatest debt to my mother, who reads everything, always.

Between the printed lines of this book are also the echoes of those living with storied scars whose narratives have yet to make it to the page. I hope this collection encourages everyone, in whatever form, to share and witness scar stories, and to appreciate those stories for all their riches.

———/———

NOTES

1. Burton is not alone among physicians. See Richard Selzer, "And if the surgeon is like a poet, then the scars you have made on countless bodies are like verses into the fashioning of which you have poured your soul. I think that if years later I were to see the trace from an old incision of mine, I would know it at once, as one recognizes his pet expressions." *Mortal Lessons: Notes on the Art of Surgery.* New York: Harcourt (1996), 94.
2. Charon, Rita. *Narrative Medicine: Honoring the Stories of Illness.* Oxford: Oxford University Press, 2006.
3. Sayantani DasGupta raises this issue in this volume as it relates to physicians and patients.

BURNED IMAGES

Jill Christman

On December 7, 1998, I mailed a letter to my father, asking him what happened on the day that my brother was burned.

I didn't think he would reply, but he did.

He wrote back—pages and pages of longhand on paper ripped from a yellow legal pad. And he began with me:

I could come up with all sorts of excuses and justifications for me not being a major part in your life, but the fact of the matter is I have not been a very good father to you primarily because of distance. . . . I feel badly that you were the child I know the least, but as I said it has mostly been the physical distance that has kept us apart, not anything between us directly.

Not anything between us directly; you were the child I know the least, my father tells me in a letter that I have asked for but never really expected to receive, in a letter whose living words I read, again and again, in a rented Tuscaloosa house, more than thirty years after my brother's skin left its indelible print on my father's palms.

I was not yet born.

———/———

My father and I barely know each other. The last time I slept under his roof, I was twenty years old, and for the first time in my life, feeling brave or reckless or grown-up or just too tired to care, I pointed my finger at him. I told him he'd never been much of a father, and he was quick with his reply: *I didn't have a father either. Your mother left me, you know.*

After that I didn't go back for almost ten years, and he began making gifts of himself. I have a stack of my father's self-portraits in a box somewhere. My father paints and repaints himself in different roles with different faces—a teacher, a man at the bottom of a pool, Martin Luther, an apple-peel head à la Escher, a man dividing at the belly like an amoeba, a turning man with three eyes or no eyes or the face of a dog—over and over he frames himself. I imagine this stack of fathers tilting upright, escaping the cardboard box one by one, frame by frame, and tottering down the hall, jerking across the hardwood floors on gilded, equilateral feet, and asking me questions: *How was school? Where is your homework? Why can't you understand that I never had a father, either?*

———/———

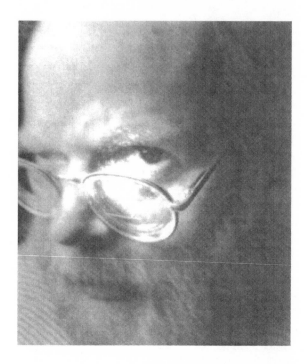

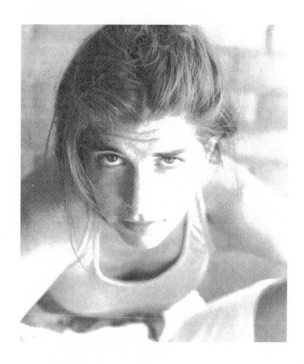

The story of Ian's burning changes like a hurt and healing body—written, erased, written over with the thick tissue of scars: coordinating palimpsests of words and flesh. Each time memory ignites, details mutate and emotion shifts: she remembers a phone call, he remembers that the diaper was on, they both remember the scream. Elements are scraped away, scribbled in, retracted, and still some pink shows through.

Today my mother breaks in: "I didn't say that—I said that there *might* have been a phone call, and you wrote it down as truth. What does your father say? He was there. I wasn't even there."

"He says he can't remember anything before Ian screamed."

"Well, how do I know, then?"

"Maybe he told you, and then he forgot."

"It was a long time ago."

"About thirty years."

"That's long. I don't even like to think about it."

"I know somebody told me once that his body was blocking the drain, and that's how the water filled up around him. How would I make something like that up?"

"I don't remember that. I never told you that."

"Maybe Ian told me."

"He doesn't remember!"

"Well, I don't know how I would make something like that up. *I mean, the baby's body is blocking the drain.*"

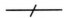

My brother carries the truth of this story on his body. I don't know how I missed this. For years I wasn't thinking hard enough. Ian has a bald spot on the top of his head, his face is burned, his shoulders are scarred; the top of his back is the worst, and then the rest of his body is unburned. The doctors stripped skin patches from his thighs when they pieced him back together, but his legs were not burned, his buttocks were not burned. There is no way Ian's body was blocking a drain while water filled up around him. His body corroborates my father's written account: *I heard a scream from the bathroom, I ran and found Ian, wearing a diaper, standing in the tub with the shower on. I turned off the water, and didn't realize how hot the water was until I picked him up and his skin came off in my hands.*

I don't remember a time when my parents were together, but I am a good listener. A quiet child, in a corner with a book open in her lap, can seem to disappear. She learns from listening, hears many things before she is old enough to understand them. When her mother's friend is fired from her job, and cries, the child knows this firing was a really bad thing and pictures the restaurant where her mother waits tables going up in flames. When she hears about the jungle warfare in Vietnam, she imagines gorillas with guns strapped to their backs and wonders what they had to fight about and where they got the guns. Sometimes it takes years for her to determine the truth behind the words. She grows into what she hears, forming images when she can, gradually, like a sheet of photographic paper soaking in developer. The pictures fill in piece by piece as she is ready to understand, taking time to color in the dark and the light spaces.

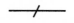

I shouldn't even be born yet.

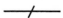

If you've ever canned peaches, you probably know that the fuzzy skin can be easily removed from the fleshy fruit by dunking the intact peach in a boiling-water bath. After a minute or so in the boiling water, the peach skin will slide off in your fingers, leaving only a shimmering, slippery globe of fruit flesh. This home-canning technique also works with tomatoes and most other skin-covered, well-fleshed bodies.

On July 22, 1966, one day after my father's twenty-third birthday, his baby boy's skin came off in his fingers like the peel of a dipped peach. This moment is at the core of our family story—some of us talk about it, some of us don't, but it is always there, like a rock at the center of a hurtling snowball.

My mother was at work, serving food to the rich at a restaurant in downtown Providence, Rhode Island—a place where she was required to bone the fish tableside so that her customers could see they were being served and protected. I wonder whether she felt the freedom of some time away from home, enjoyed being out with other people—even at work. Or whether she worried about her baby at home, wished she could be there to give him his bedtime bath, turn the pages of a book, nurse him to sleep.

In this story, my mother is only twenty-one, a young wife, mother, and waitress. She couldn't walk through her art school graduation the previous spring because, at the that time, she was had been nine months pregnant. Her new name is Martha Ingraham Christman. She is pretty in a way that might be called wholesome: dark curly hair, deep-brown eyes, a confident Ingraham nose, breasts that are full and round with milk for her baby. Martha is quick to smile, always ready to comfort, and practiced in the dual roles of caretaker and peacekeeper (in 1966, her father is an alcoholic, her teenage brother is a drug addict, and nobody has started talking about codependency). At only twenty-one years of age, she is a nurturing mother, an attentive waitress, and she is trying to be a wife. Any kind of wife.

She was young when she married my father. "Too young," she tells me again and again. "I didn't want to marry him. I just wanted to live with him for a summer, out on the Vineyard. But Grammy and Grandfather wouldn't let me. They said if I wanted to live with him, I had to marry him. You have to understand, things were different then. I thought I was doing the right thing. I thought I had to marry your father because I slept with him. I even thought I loved him because I had sex with him. I didn't know you could have the one without the other—that's how naïve I was. So I married him. And I'm glad. Because I have you." My mother tells me that my father didn't actually give her the engagement ring. His mother did, because she liked my mother and had decided that she would make a good wife for her son. It was really as simple as that, according to my mother. Or maybe not. *My father's letter breaks into the narrative, erases, rewrites: No woman could ever be good enough for me in my mother's eyes. She didn't approve of Marty until we were separated. Then she was perfect in comparison.* (The story of the ring cannot be corroborated by my father's mother. She has been dead for more than twenty years.)

"Your Grammy Sarah was a difficult mother for your father to have," my mother explains. "She was very controlling. I mean, an amazing woman, and I admit that I might have been more infatuated with Sarah than I was with your father. She threw the best parties on the Vineyard, you know. She'd be wild even now. But definitely a difficult woman to have for a mother."

So, my mother was young, still an undergraduate at the Rhode Island School of Design, when she began a life as wife and mother—a hasty June wedding, nine months of pregnancy spent sprinting from reeking painting studios to the bathroom to throw up, twenty-eight hours of labor, and thirteen short months of healthy baby boy later—and my mother is about to arrive at the instant she will look back on thirty years later as the single most defining moment of her life. It is around 8 p.m., and Martha is pouring Chardonnay, rotating her wrist to stop the flow of wine without a drip, and highlighting the evening's specials for a couple at table number four. Another waitress touches her arm and tells her that she'll take the order. There's a phone call. An emergency. The baby. That is how I see my mother on the night that my brother was burned: content, busy, engaged in normal restaurant bustle, until that tap on the arm. . . . But nothing has happened yet. Her husband is home with baby Ian in this story, and everything is fine.

My father is sitting in the kitchen of their first-floor apartment in Providence, talking on the telephone. I can picture him there, with his bare feet up on the round oak table. Above the table hangs an enormous oil painting, five-by-eight feet at least, of a mass of people in a crowded place, maybe a New York City subway station, and there is an unsmiling woman in a pale pink, formfitting dress. The signature in the lower left-hand corner of the painting is an illegible scrawl. Translated, the artist's name reads: Pete Christman.

(This has not always been my father's name. He was born Adrian Fryers Jr., because that's what his father wanted it to be, but his mother always called him "Pete," after her reckless brother, a Yale graduate who left a good job on the northeastern seaboard and struck out for parts unknown, ending up living a cowboy's life on a ranch in Montana until he died in his thirties of a ruptured appendix. Pete. To my knowledge, my father met his biological father only twice—*I was a product of World War II*, my father tells me in the same long letter. Patrilineally speaking, my name should be Jill Fryers. But then Grammy Sarah went ahead and married—and eventually divorced—a man named Bill Christman. When the man left, the name stayed.)

But this is a story about Pete Christman and his baby, Ian, in 1966. As Pete listens to the voice coming through the receiver, he is probably plucking a hair from the knuckle on his big toe, wetting the root of the hair with the tip of his tongue, and examining it over the top of his glasses. He repeats this ritual—pluck, lick, examination—with hair all over his body: beard hairs, head hairs, mustache hairs.

I don't know who he's on the phone with, but I pretend that it's his mother. She wants to know if his birthday package arrived, how he liked the canned herring, whether the tan corduroys fit, how the baby is doing. When his mother asks about the baby, Pete notices that Ian is no longer in the kitchen with him. Perhaps he's in the bedroom playing with the dog. The corduroys are a bit snug, but the herring is delicious, had it for lunch with bagels and cream cheese. The poor man's lox, my father tells her, laughing; he likes to play the part of the struggling art student even though he attended an exclusive prep school, even though he knows that when his mother dies, she will leave him more than enough to be comfortable.

Where is the baby who is supposed to be in this story?

After the phone call—a detail once provided by my mother, although, of course, the herring and the corduroys and even the line about lox are fictional props in the role of authentic detail—the story gets fuzzy, except for the sound of Ian's scream and the hiss of squirting water. This is where Pete's memory clicks in. The baby isn't in the kitchen. He swings his feet off the table, stands up, and runs down the hall to the bathroom. He hasn't yet turned the corner to the bathroom. For a second or two more he is a husband and father in good standing. The baby is screaming.

For twenty-nine years, until last month's letter from my father, this is the shared family memory, this is what Pete sees when he comes around the corner and into the bathroom: The baby's body is blocking the drain in the bathtub. Steaming water is spurting out of the faucet. Water is rising around the baby. The baby is boiling.

But now we know that it isn't the faucet, it's the shower. And the baby hasn't fallen. He is standing solid on his two small feet. He is standing and screaming. Tilt into my father's version, lean into the past tense of his memory:

I found Ian, wearing a diaper, standing in the tub with the shower on. I turned off the water, and didn't realize how hot the water was until I picked him up and his skin came off in my hands.

This jibes with the shared story. Pete's first instinct is to grab the baby out of the water, and he does this, and that's when Ian's skin slides off into his hands. *I have a mental snapshot of this which I carry with me to this day.* Pete doesn't know yet that the baby has burns on more than 80 percent of his body, but he can see that his son's face is melting away like the wax on a candle. His baby is glowing red—he is a hot coal, a boiled lobster, a peeled peach. This baby boy looks like many things, steaming and unconscious and sticking in his father's arms, but he does not look human.

I have a mental snapshot of this which I carry with me to this day. I knew [he] was seriously hurt, but had no idea of what my then new family was about to face. I grabbed a clean sheet and then a towel, wrapped Ian in it and ran upstairs to the second floor to find someone to drive us to the emergency room.

The thermostat was turned up too high on the water heater in their ground-floor apartment. Maybe my father will read the warning above the dial on the water heater when he returns home from the hospital that night: WATER AT OR ABOVE 125 DEGREES IS SCALDING, AND IS EXTREMELY DANGEROUS TO THE VERY YOUNG AND THE VERY OLD. Then he will curse himself for not reading the warning earlier. And he will curse himself for never even thinking about the temperature of the water coming out of the faucet—didn't he always just add cold? But mostly he will curse himself for not being attentive, for not knowing how carefully a baby needs to be watched. He will curse himself for everything he did that night, any one moment of which, if altered, might have changed the course of events that had brought him to that moment when his son's skin came apart in his fingers. And when he is done cursing, he will begin again. He will curse himself until he has to leave to deaden the sound of his own cursing, and then, a letter written thirty-four years after the burning to a critical daughter who had not been born in time to live through that day, will read like a confession:

I guess the first things to be dealt with are facts to answer your questions
with. Then I will try to remember as accurately as possible what happened. It
is interesting that I can't at this point remember what I was doing on July 22,
1966, until I heard Ian's scream. You are supposed to forget the actual event
and not what led up to it. That summer I had just graduated from RISD and
was working painting a factory during the days, and then we would have
a change of the guard and I would take care of Ian while Marty worked as
a waitress. Ian was 13 mo. old, just beginning to walk and into everything.
After seeing five children go through this period of development I know that
they must be watched every second, but at that point I had worked in a hot
factory all day and was I guess more interested in relaxing with a cold beer
than watching Ian the way I should have. . . . I can't remember what was
happening before Ian was hurt. I know I carry a lot of guilt about my part in
Ian's accident, and I have suppressed key details.

There are pieces that will always be missing from the story of my
brother's burning. Ian says he has no memory of that night, and so he will
hold the gaps of the story—how he got into the tub, why he turned on the
water, what that kind of pain feels like—deep in the grooves of the scars on
his body for the rest of his life.

After my brother's skin slides from his body and onto the hands of his
father, the story is less immediate. Time slows down and returns obediently
to the past tense and the frame of my mother's voice. She says that my
father got the upstairs neighbor, although nobody can remember his name.
(But perhaps someone can—*I think his name was Jim,* my father says now.)
Somehow all three of them—the neighbor now known as Jim, the father,
and the burned baby—got to the hospital, and that is when the other
waitress touched my mother's arm: "I'll take it. You have a phone call. An
emergency. The baby."

My mother drove to the emergency room in her waitressing uniform
and took over the story. She talks still about those months in the hospital
with Ian whenever she wants to make someone understand that she knows
how it feels to grieve and sweat and pray and wait.

The doctors wouldn't allow my parents to see my brother that first night,
so they went home to sleep. My mother says that she didn't know how bad
it was: "My fear was that he would have scarring. Not that he might not
live. I had no idea. No idea. Before the doctors let me see him, they told
me that I had to realize that Ian's condition was 'grave.' They'd cut in a trach
tube, but he still was having trouble breathing. The swelling was terrible.
The doctors told us he only had a one-in-ten chance—to live, not to die.
One in ten." Here, the stories mesh, in that indelible, corroborated statistic:
At that point we were told that Ian had a 10 percent chance of survival. I

think both Marty and I grew up at that moment.

"When I saw him for the first time, I didn't even know what I was looking at. He was just this little, red, pumping, swollen-up thing on green sheets. He looked like a baby orangutan. He was bright red, but it was the swelling that made him look so strange. An orangutan, or a space creature. But he was my baby, and he was beautiful. Those green sheets *were* ugly. They were special ones that were supposed to reduce the risk of infection—that was the big fear—and not stick to him as much. Everything stuck to him." And, of course, I always want to know if she was mad at my father for being there when it happened. She always says no. "I was more overwhelmed than mad. I was so young, practically a kid myself. We were both young. We were *all* young. And something like that will certainly change your perspective on life."

I think both Marty and I grew up at that moment. Our beautiful child was wrapped in bandages with tubes coming out of the bundle. Everything was hospital clean and clinical.

Ian was in the burn unit for more than four months. My mother slept on a cot in his room. At some point, my father moved to Syracuse, New York, to begin graduate school:

Ian continued to improve. He still looked pretty bad. There were problems of weaning him off of the trach tube in his throat, but this was finally successfully accomplished. He was out of immediate danger. Ian was going to live but would still have to remain in the hospital another two months.

I had been accepted to graduate school scheduled to start in the fall. I was willing to stay in Providence, but we decided that I should move to Syracuse and start working on my M.F.A. I came back to Providence on several occasions with the plan that Marty and Ian would move to Syracuse when he got out of the hospital. As the time approached for the big move, Marty decided that she wasn't going to Syracuse, and we split up.

After my brother's burning, both my parents met other people: a man and a woman who didn't think about the accident every minute of every day, a man and a woman who were both able to take hot showers without smelling the boiled flesh of a baby. The story gets hazy here, but I know there were other loves, and then some talk of reconciliation.

"I went back to him when your brother was three," my mother says. "It was Christmas! Maybe I was in the holiday spirit, maybe it seemed like your brother should be with his father at Christmas. I wanted to have another baby so that Ian would have a little brother or sister. I wanted to have another baby that matched."

———/———

Afterword to "Burned Images," March 2015:

This morning, when I told my ten-year-old daughter Ella that I was writing about scars, she ran to get her battered copy of *Harry Potter and the Sorcerer's Stone* and read me a passage from the beginning when Dumbledore, McGonagall, and Hagrid convene on Privet Drive to leave Harry on the doorstep. Fifteen-month-old Harry, of course, has just received the wound that will become that most notorious of literary scars: the red lightning bolt carved in his soft forehead by an evil so deep it mustn't be named. Because Harry's scar will bear permanent witness to the attack that killed his parents, Professor McGonagall suggests they might remove it to spare Harry the pain of the mark. Dumbledore disagrees, arguing for the utility of Harry's scar; after all, hadn't the scar-map of the London Underground above Dumbledore's own knee served him well all these years?

Scars are complicated for those of us who bear them—and let's face it, that's pretty much the entire human race. Scars are a history written on the body, permanent marks that remain after the trauma and the healing, and like all enduring texts, their meaning shifts with the reader and the time of the reading. Fourteen years ago, when I wrote "Burned Images" as chapter one in the memoir of the first thirty years of my life (*Darkroom: A Family Exposure*, University of Georgia Press, 2002), I was not yet a mother. Writing the story of my family's original scarring, I worked hard to turn the lens, see the different angles—the guilt-ridden father whose negligence opened the door to the accident, the forgiving and devastated mother who got the news of her baby's burning at the restaurant where she worked, the baby who wore the soft skin that *came off in his [father's] fingers like the peel of a dipped peach*, even the unborn little sister who was me, carrying a tragedy she came too late to witness.

But when I wrote that peach, my skin hadn't yet expanded to hold my own babies and the new fear that comes with them. Now, I can't even sit still to finish reading the chapter I wrote all those years ago. I have to run down the dark basement stairs to check the dial on the hot water heater. This is not a metaphor. This is my life.

I wrote "Burned Images" when I was a young woman thinking about her own scars—all of them psychological but for three: the sweet crescent moon on my right knee carved by a surprise sliver of glass on a dirt hill when I was seven, an inch-long ridge on the outer edge of my thumb cut in by a Cuisinart blade submerged beneath the bubbles (stupid, stupid, stupid), and two ghostly parallel lines on my left wrist that are part of a story I long ago wanted to write on my own flesh with the sharpest blade I could find. (*Please don't let Ella ever know this kind of pain.* And yet how can I protect her? I know I cannot.) The stories I need to tell are so different now, stories written over stories, stories upon stories, histories piled up for excavation—on our pages, in our hearts, on our skin. Conduct an inventory of your own scars. Do you see how the narratives layer and shift?

The story of Ian's burning changes like a hurt and healing body—written, erased, written over with the thick tissue of scars: coordinating palimpsests of words and flesh. I remember how I wanted to use that word—*palimpsests*— and how perfect it seemed to describe my brother's skin with its smooth, hairless valleys and rising peaks, the healed skin of his rewritten topography as hard and smooth as lava rock. After the scalding water made its mark, the surgeons moved in with their own instruments balanced like drafting pencils in their elegant fingers. On Ian's thigh, for example, they drew a perfect rectangle, a sheet of notebook paper, peeling back the clean layers and grafting them onto those places on his back and shoulders where the water hadn't left enough. When he was twelve or thirteen, moving into puberty and literally outgrowing his own skin, the burn doctors cut a wedge from Ian's bicep to make room for the developing muscles. I remember thinking of the wedges of iceberg lettuce our mother would give us with bleu cheese dressing. The doctors left the wound open, and when my mother changed the gauze dressings, I stole a peek inside my brother's body. The idea was that the skin would grow back over.

The doctors did what they could, and still, Ian's skin was pulled and stretched in those places the hot water had hit like nothing the neighborhood kids had ever seen before, and yet—and here is the story I want to remember—on hot days my brother would pull off his shirt, throw it onto the sand, and let them look. Unashamed. If new kids came around, strangers, sometimes they would stare and say, "What's wrong with your brother? Why is his skin all . . . *bumpy*?" And I would shrug, tell them he'd been burned. *I don't even notice*, I'd say. And it was true.

At readings, people often want to know how my brother Ian is doing, and the answer is: *Just fine. He's doing great.* He'll turn fifty next summer, which means he's existed nearly forty-nine years, all the years he's known, really, in this rewritten body of his. He lives in the Atlanta suburbs, works as the creative director for a medical website company, makes art and music, serves faithfully and well as a husband, and as father to two beautiful girls. It's more complicated than this, of course. He needs to lose some weight. He could probably stand to cut down on the cocktails. This summer he sent me a photo on my phone of his new beard, a goatee cut in just right in those places he can grow hair on his face. Ian's first real beard. *Looking sharp*, I texted back. Ian's scars are a part of who he is and what he survived. He took that ten percent chance and ran with it all the way into his lucky life.

For Ella's ninth birthday, we threw her a Hogwarts party, and after breaking through the red table cloth I'd painted with bricks to resemble Platform 9 ¾, the children lined up and I zigged lightning-bolt scars in red marker above all the left eyebrows in the teeming Great Hall, each child a gleeful Potter-esque survivor of something evil, grinning as they ran off to brew foaming truth serum in potions class.

This morning, Ella helped me to begin this afterword, pointing with her finger to Dumbledore's wise counsel. Scars remind us how to *live*. "Yes," I said, accepting the book she held out and kissing her smooth cheek. "That's true. Thank you." Ella ran off to play with her little brother Henry while I turned back to my work with the words she'd left behind and my daily prayer. *Please keep them safe.*

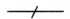

A THOUSAND STITCHES OF PINK SILK

Annie Tucker

when i was still a kid we learned that
my older sister's spine had been collapsing
helix twisting
contours rising
crooked

next to her at the dinner table, i liked to rest my hand on her growing
hump
it seemed to swell out into my palm, breathing—
another new curve that i didn't have yet.

but she was ashamed and in pain,
her mood growing ever darker. she had to stop doing
the things she loved: bike trips, gymnastics competitions.
as she started to hide behind her long black hair
i started tagging along in the back seat,
from chiropractors to energy aligners to specialty surgeons, i sat
quiet in the corner of our library as she lay on copper screens
i watched from her bed as she velco-strapped herself into complicated
braces,
like before when i would sit on the toilet in the bathroom
as she hooked her bra, did her makeup to go out.

i went to visit her in the hospital,
after they had sliced her open and fused her spine and
put in the harrington rods:
parallel lines of stainless steel
to give her support, to keep her straight.
she lay flat, she moaned in pain.
when she rolled over
through the parting at the back of her gown
i could see the scar
a horizon
that started under her slim nape
and reached between the newly muted swells of her
shoulder blades to come gliding through
the shallows of the small of her back

finally resting right above her tailbone.
at the top it looked like a thin line of ink
traced across the surface
then as it descended it also widened and rose up
a thick pink silky ridge
that looked like a seam, as if it was not made of skin
but of the thousand stitches of fine thread
they had used to sew her back together.

after weeks of her recovery
my mother was exhausted and
my grandmother came to stay.
she took us out to dinner.
as the appetizers arrived
my sister burst into tears
she hated her body
and she hated her scar
my mother and i froze
but with a casual glamour
my grandmother said :

don't worry, honey

some
day
a
man
will
kiss
that
scar
up
and
down

and my mother gasped

and i choked
on my bread
with envy.

SOMETHING FAITHFUL

Marcus Cafagña

I can't imagine the seasons
of ruffles and turtlenecks until she
allowed it to be seen,

my aunt Eleanor's throat scarred
by the blade of a knife.
But now it's the itch of healing

at family gatherings. In something
low cut the scar is a deep red
valley into which I cannot

look. Still, she's never accused
my cousin of madness or hated
the heroin he tried to kick

with Quaaludes. She only ducks
her chin at times, says
it shows a mother and son

can live separate
lives since a scar is something
faithful, a way her skin

will never give him up.

—/—

TISSUE

Erin Wood

I place my daughter's skin over my skin like layers of tissue paper, translucent layers, her scar story over my scar story. I hold the layers up against the light. Behind them, shadows move.

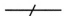

I think of her skin. Her skin of my skin. Her first skin.

Once they had her stabilized, shortly after she was born, nurses and doctors wheeled her into the room where I had pushed her from my body with dread.

There she lay in the basinet, on display. Her skin: fuchsia and furious, reflectively taut, spotted in purple and black. Even the palms of her hands—the size of the tips of my thumbs—bruised. Someone said she weighed 640 grams, which translates to 1 pound and 7 ounces if you round up.

Her head was little larger than a misshapen racquet ball, one of the blue and pink and white striped hats that they put on all the newborns at the hospital was the size of a small blanket under her head. Her legs and arms were pinky fingers splayed out from her body, her feet long like rabbits' feet at the ends of legs that were nothing more than bone and skin.

How were we supposed to keep her alive? Her father and I examined her for familiar parts and shapes and markings, searched for something we could interpret. But we could not understand, this scene so unlike anything we'd ever imagined that we couldn't even determine how to respond. There was no cooing, no holding—just a settling sense that we were powerless. When we nodded to her nurses, her still, red body was wheeled away to wherever it was in the hospital they would take her to do whatever it is they do to save the lives of babies like her. *Were there any other babies like her?*

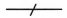

I think of my first skin. My skin that would someday become her skin. I rewrite its story, a story that also began with a baby in a bassinet. A story that also began with a mother in fear for the life of her baby.

My first skin, pink and plump and firm, covering organs that twenty-four hours later doctors discovered were not all fully functioning. Meconium that did not pass. An intussusception of the colon. A prolapse. A telescoping of skin into skin that created an obstruction. A dire emergency for a newborn that in 2014 is treated simply by passing air through the digestive tract but in 1978 was treated by surgery to cut away the telescoped skin and join the remaining tissues. My surgeon grandfather must have been pacing outside the OR with my parents, understanding the stakes, likely hiding his understanding from the rest of my family.

The first cut of the scalpel on a small, smooth field, the slicing away, the carving out, the rejoining of tissues, clean edge against clean edge, my life made possible in the healing of that gap. And then a colostomy. And then a mother with an empty belly forced to leave her baby in the care of nurses and doctors.

———+———

Twenty-four (or was it forty-eight?) hours after her birth, lying in a bed in a wing of the hospital separate from the Neonatal Intensive Care Unit, I was still in no hurry to see my baby.

The statistics on the document that I had hidden away in a zippered pocket of my purse admonished me: 23 weeks <500 grams, 5% chance of *intact survival. *23 weeks >500 grams, 21% chance of* *intact survival. 23 weeks + 640 grams= 21% chance. The asterisk linked to a definition for intact: "Survival without severe brain hemorrhage or severe eye disease." I couldn't remember whether I had historically considered myself lucky, but the answer seemed to matter. I celebrated myself for the extra fat and calories I'd consumed in countless Haagen-Dazs milkshakes during pregnancy that were now translating into a 16% better chance that our baby would live.

From that bed in the hospital, I read and reread the document, "Outcome Concerns in the Borderline Viable Infant SVHSP 5798 (0310)." It was numbered so that it could be found easily among files in an office, a bar code at the bottom so it could be scanned when given to parents. I was once a practicing lawyer. I knew this was the kind of thing that lawyers do. I was thankful not to have been the kind of lawyer that would have to draft a form like this.

> "There does appear to be a threshold of gestational age below which there are not survivors. That threshold appears to be **23 completed weeks.**"

In bold was "23 completed weeks," just like that. We knew the precise date because I had in vitro fertilization. She was 23 weeks and 6 days.

"At <24 weeks with good accurate dates, it is permissible to request '*comfort care*' only."

Also in bold was "comfort care," apparently so that grieving, desperate, confused parents could cling to that phrase when they got lost in the sea of words and 9 point font. We could have requested comfort care, and it would have been understood. Sanctioned even. But we chose resuscitation. The document went on to list potential calamities.

Reasons for poor survival and poor outcome in the 22–24 week gestation baby include:
- Poor lung function due to very small and incompletely formed lungs
- Heart failure from a heart too weak to pump oxygen-rich blood to vital organs
- Kidney failure which often leads to no urine production
- Intestines prone to poor digestive function and rupture
- A very immature immune system that does not protect the baby from overwhelming infection
- Very immature blood vessels in the brain which lead to brain hemorrhages in 35–50% of babies in this group, leading to stroke, brain death, cerebral palsy, or the need for a shunt drainage tube
- Very immature blood vessels in the retina of the eye which can lead to retinal detachment and possible blindness

"Let her go," one reading would seem to suggest, to whisper even. And then in the next I would find the slight, if quickly vacillating, hope of *21%! That's almost a quarter of babies like her! Or maybe it is closer to a fifth. . . .*
In the hospital bed I was reading from a copy, but each day during the preceding week, my husband and I had been asked to sign and re-sign this form.

Based on a discussion of the above information, I understand the outcome statistics and possibility for poor outcome in survivors in the borderline viability group. For my baby I desire:
- Compassionate Comfort Care.
- Resuscitation with ongoing involvement in decision making if care becomes futile.

For Isabel, we chose resuscitation. For her twin brother, we had chosen compassionate comfort care. But in the end, the choice regarding her brother was made for us when his heart had stopped beating in utero.

I had folded and unfolded and refolded the sheet of paper until it was divided into quarters, the ink worn away at the creases. I needed to make sure that I understood. That I had the facts straight. I tried to think like a lawyer.

But there in that bed I was no longer a lawyer and not much of a mother. I had never been a statistician, but I knew statistics were utterly subjective, prone to manipulation. If the statistics happened to be correct, perhaps it was better not to go to her until it was determined whether or not she would be among the 21%. *But when would they know? Days? Weeks? Months? Jesus Christ, years?* What would I find in her room at the end of the hallways that twisted and turned through the NICU? It was a mystery no document could divine.

After what must have been a hopeful reading, I finally grew brave enough to search for her. My husband had gone before me several times, so he knew the way, pushing my wheelchair through various security checkpoints until we finally reached her room. I recall my pause at that door, that sliding glass door behind which a curtain drew down between us, that door that I can see if I close my eyes even now. I contemplated marking the moment I stood in that doorway as one of those moments we all look back on after something terrible happens, those precious seconds which—if you went left instead of right, if you stopped a breathbeat sooner—could divert you from disaster. That door extended to me an offer to turn back.

But I entered. At the center of the room, she was sealed in a plastic box under an otherworldly blue light. Her limbs were stretched out in four directions like a pinned specimen. *Weren't babies supposed to curl up?* She wore a mask over her eyes, which we would come to know as her "Biliglasses," the coverings that protected her eyes from the Bilirubin lights that were helping to prevent jaundice. *Kidney failure which often leads to no urine production.*

I knew this was not what a baby should look like—unmoving, mouth propped permanently open by a ventilator, tethered to twenty machines that were reading and assessing and pumping and beeping—but I knew that she was our baby. At least the facts pointed to her being our baby, and the sign outside her door had read "BG Wood." She was a baby girl with our last name, and the first name we had chosen for her months before. Isabel. My mother's name.

She had been inside my body, but I could not keep her there. I could not keep her brother there and now he was gone. She was in her surrogate womb, a womb that was supposed to do what my body failed to do. Her *isolette*. The iterations of that word were not lost on me. I had gone to her side and yet I did not dare in those first days to place my hands through the portholes that would have connected our worlds. I could not hold her close. I could have touched her palm with my gloved finger, but I chose not to. I had no way of knowing her, and I wasn't sure that it was safe even to search for some way to connect.

She was so separate from our life, living in that small, electric box deep within the winding corridors of that enormous hospital, so tiny in comparison to the immense building it seemed she could be misplaced. And who was making sure that she wouldn't go missing? Once I got my bearings, I became suspicious of the only people who knew how to keep her alive. Where did they go to college, to nursing school, to grad school, to med school? What were the credentials of her nutritionist, her respiratory therapist?

But my suspicions did not give me a voice. I did not yet know how to be her advocate, her champion. I only raged inside when nurses laughed as if something—anything—was worth laughing about. I learned that if she grew cold, even by a degree, she would utilize all her energy to raise her body temperature rather than to heal. The womb and the isolette do this for babies so that they can dedicate their resources to other things. When some therapist left her portholes open too long, causing the cool air of her room to seep in and lower her body temperature, the isolette shouted with a vicious DING! that resonated at a place I never knew existed deep within my chest. When I heard the sound, I tried to disappear into the corner, I crunched down and cowered. I said nothing.

I did not know how to love her. I did not understand what she needed from me, nor what I could give her. Maybe the people who cared for these babies knew better. It was the ultimate defeat. Mother does not know best—I was turning the cliché on its end.

Little by little, I got stronger, leaving my wheelchair to visit her on foot, walking slowly. Then picking up the pace, rediscovering my normal gait, the pain in my gut and between my legs lessening. And finally, I was released from the hospital. My husband and I went home with my empty belly, our empty car, our empty hearts.

The only efforts I could think of making felt futile. I pumped milk for her that she could not consume, placing it in little plastic containers to go in a NICU freezer. I cried into soft, pink clothes she could not wear. I closed the door to the half-decorated nursery that I imagined she might never see. I would re-learn how to grind through the day, how to park my car, to go through the lobby, to push the elevator button, to sterilize myself, to put on a gown, to stand next to her box and watch her as she lay still as a stone, the only signs of life coming from the machines that monitored every aspect of her. I had the sense that a mother should do something more for her baby. *But what?*

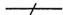

When I was one and then two and then three, I had more surgeries. More surgeons' fingers guided scalpels horizontally across my middle, opening my body in an attempt to solve the problems of my digestion. More incisions. More scarring. A vertical incision. And then, a diagnosis. Though it surely brought more worries, it must have been a relief to my parents to have a label: Hirschsprung's Disease, the diagnosis handed down from a famed doctor in Memphis. I was to be the youngest child yet diagnosed, and he was to be in journals. A surgery to remove a substantial part of my colon. A post-surgical biopsy, negative for Hirschsprung's Disease. Fingers pointed to the radiologist who read the pre-surgical slide, to the doctor who would now not be in journals. A lawsuit. A jurisdictional technicality ending the lawsuit. A colostomy removed and a child left with bowel incontinence.

Medicine had both saved and shattered my life. Kids made fun of me and didn't want to be my friends. I had my suspicions about the kids who did; I knew they must have been hiding secrets of their own. If we were friends long enough, my suspicions were confirmed when I stayed at their houses: ticks full of blood that crawled from under the house where dogs slept in filthy pits, a father who threw shoeboxes at his daughter's face, a mother who never ate and danced in the storage shed in her pointe shoes until her toes bled.

Like the friends I felt lucky to have, I lived in shame, certain there was something I could do to change what was happening to me but never sure what that something was. My parents' divorce and my father's cruelty only made matters worse, and soon I began hiding in my room on the days I stayed with my father, pounding on my thighs until they bruised, trying to make myself pay.

I don't remember being ashamed of the marks on my body, marks that ran (and still run) in the four cardinal directions, dividing my body in quarters. But I was barely surviving the shame of what they signified—the evidence of my body's failures. There were plenty of reasons to hide, to change clothes in dark corners at summer camp, to keep kids from seeing those scars and coming for what I needed to keep from them—my hideous story.

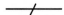

By the time Isabel was about a week old and still under a pound and a half, we had battled a "Grade II" brain bleed. *Very immature blood vessels in the brain which lead to brain hemorrhages in 35–50% of babies in this group, leading to stroke, brain death, cerebral palsy, or the need for a shunt drainage tube.* Then early one morning while having coffee at home, we got the worst call imaginable from the hospital—*You need to get here right away,* her nurse practitioner Ramona's voice. They only call in life and death situations because they know the sight of the phone number alone on the caller id is enough to send any NICU parent into hysterics.

An immediate ligation of her patent ductus arteriosis was necessary; her lungs were filling with fluid. She was drowning. We anxiously signed forms listing all that could go wrong, including damage to the nerves of the left vocal fold—a detail that hardly seemed to matter in the face of the life-saving surgery. A detail that would only become relevant months later. The surgeon went through her back, through her ribcage, to ligate the fetal heart valve that normally closes at birth, but in preemies allows blood and fluid to fill up their lungs, putting their lives in jeopardy. *Poor lung function due to very small and incompletely formed lungs; Heart failure from a heart too weak to pump oxygen-rich blood to vital organs.*

After the surgery, her heart became stronger, there was less fluid to remove from her lungs, her monitors' distressing *DING!* happened less often. She had once again cheated death.

Then, her skin began to slough, sliding from what should have been its hold against anything that touched it—her diaper, the hospital-issue newborn blankets that covered her bed, the foam cuffs that held her IVs straight, the ventilator where it laid across her lower lip, the electrodes that monitored her vitals, her own skin where it met other skin on her body, like in the creases of her ankles. After her skin slid away, what remained wept and oozed.

The voices that tried to give us answers were echoes in a strange, reverberating chamber. I heard wisps of information, but most were lost into the ether. *When they come so early, this can happen*, they said. For 17 weeks longer, for over 4 months more, she should have been floating freely, turning easily, carefree inside the lightless goop of my body.

At this point in the womb, only one or two layers of skin are formed. Adults have nine, they said. One or two layers of skin, thin as tissue paper. This is why, when the leads that were monitoring her heart rate and breathing were removed, they took her skin with them. This is why without those precious layers, she had little to protect herself and developed an infection. *A very immature immune system that does not protect the baby from overwhelming infection.* Without more time, she had few defenses.

Then a savvy thought from her nurse practitioner, Ramona: *Maybe the burn unit has some ideas.*

The burn unit buttered her with special salve and applied special gauze generally reserved for burn victims, giving her a slippery barrier. She shone under the lights that made what was left of her skin a window into the blue and purple of capillaries and the white of bones. With no fat beneath it, her skin was translucent; we were looking into her body. There were the veins at the surface, pumping blood at visible intervals, there were the ribs at the surface, encasing a heart that struggled to beat. Ghosts were there in her skin, taunting us by revealing all that was wrong with her body; we could see everything, but we could do nothing.

The nurses tried to do less, to touch and poke as little as possible through the portholes that were the barrier between her isolette and the open air of the NICU. Doing less meant a greater likelihood of maintaining the rainforest atmosphere inside her isolette—keeping the humidity high and the temperature constant.

She will be scarred all over her body from this infection, they said. *And no matter how old they are, you can always tell a preemie by the track marks on their hands and feet.*

But scarring was the least of our worries then. Germs were everywhere, magnified, propelled through the air, travelling from baby to baby on nurses' scrubs, under all of our fingernails, in all of our breath, waiting. Every handshake was a threat, every surface and every body a transport for contagion, every person who coughed a reason to leave a room. There was little more than wet tissue paper holding her body in, keeping every horror out, somehow bearing up the weight of our lives.

I do not have to try very hard to remember what was nearly upon us, that hot breath at the back of our necks. Sometimes, when I dare to peer back in time, and if I recognize that I am feeling weak, I try to concentrate all my strength on not remembering.

Somehow, by some power of medicine or some grace or some stroke of luck, the shadows departed her body and her infection healed. Her weeping skin transformed into a molting sheath, little yellow flakes each of which we were told were a bit of evidence that things were looking up. I was permitted to hold her hot little molting body against my chest. Two nurses were necessary to tuck her into my un-buttoned Oxford shirt with all her cords and her vent, to position her head comfortably. They said that my heartbeat would calm her. I didn't think that was possible since my heartbeat was audible, filling my ears with the sound of a galloping herd. But first for a few minutes, and then weeks later for all-day, marathon "Kangaroo Care" sessions, we began to know each other. I learned her pizza dough smell. I felt how her body relaxed when she heard Helen Jane Long on the piano. Her vitals responded to my proximity. We began to feel more like a unit, like a mother and her baby even. Finally, finally, there was something I could do for her.

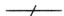

My mother's heart surely broke for me, just as all mother's hearts must break for their ill babies, each of the nine times we learned I would need abdominal surgery.

Scar tissue. We so often think of it as what is visible. But in my case, that is less than half the story. Turn my body inside out and what you'd see would make the deep, directional scars on the surface of my belly seem trivial. Inside, dark caverns of adhesions have led to obstructions, more surgeries, more adhesions. My organs are no longer movable, no longer distinct entities, but great masses battened one to the next by scar tissue. In some ways I am better—the shame of my childhood incontinence resolved by a gifted surgeon and family friend when I was in junior high. But the shortcomings of my body still offer their sufferings.

My last surgery was to remove my fallopian tubes—those first cuts and those mistaken cuts and all the cuts that followed them culminating in that operating room, on that table, robbing my ability to naturally become pregnant, perhaps even leading to the premature rupture of membranes around our baby boy, perhaps shaping the story of Isabel's scars. The scalpel extends far beyond the skin that it first cuts, layering tissue over tissue, story over story.

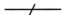

Near the end of our 128 day NICU stay, my husband and I asked for a consult with the pediatric dermatologist. Perhaps we were turning our thoughts to surface concerns like scar tissue and how she might cope with the damaged skin that covers her chest once she entered adolescence in order to turn them away from thoughts like what if, once we get her home, her home oxygen machine stops working or she stops breathing or her heart stops beating.

Whatever the reasons, we wanted advice on how we might ameliorate the damage to her chest or what options might be available to her someday should she be bothered by her scars and choose to pursue those options. The doctor said that over time, the topography of her scar tissue will change, that it will grow with her. I know from my own history of scarring that when he says they will grow with her, he means they will grow larger. His best advice was to lotion her up daily, that time would tell, and that there may be treatments available to her in fifteen or twenty years—ones we can't yet imagine.

During the intervening two and a half years, we have waited and watched. We have had the luxury of what our favorite NICU doc called "the tincture of time." Month by month, her oxygen canula which used to connect her to the canister with a 50-foot tube we dragged all around the house, her monitors, her leg braces, her bottles of thickened formula, have come and gone, leaving her tethered to nothing except the skin that holds her in its care.

The now large squares of skin where the leads were removed are thinner than the rest of the skin on her body. Through that thin tissue, I imagine I am looking at the very map of her survival—the veins that carried the blood, even the donor blood that was transfused a dozen times, to all her organs, strengthening them cell by cell, building up the layers of her skin.

At one point, we feared that she would have no nipple on the right side of her chest. The area where her nipple seemed as if it should be looked exactly the same as the rest of the scar tissue. But, one day a pink dot differentiated itself, and we were relieved for her. As impossibly strange as it is to think of your toddler as a future sexual being, there is the question: what might a lover think? Will the lovers she meets someday tell her she is more beautiful for her scars? Or will their shock and their cruel words make her feel distressed, even ugly or ruined? Of course we hope she chooses her lovers wisely, and rejects with confidence those who fall short.

As much as I would love to boast that the confidence that led me to accept my own scars came from within, the truth (as much as we ever have one) is that it hangs on the words of a college boyfriend—a 6' 5", 285 pound football player who grew up on the streets, in a gang. When he saw my abdomen, and told me my scars were cool, I believed him. I believed him and for me, everything in my life turned around that belief, the shadows and the shame diminished, and I became able to look people in the eyes and feel that I was worthy. I hope that Isabel doesn't need to hear such words from the mouth of another to believe that she is worthy, but if she does need them, I hope that the words are hanging in the air for her, just waiting to be heard.

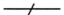

These days, Isabel is, as her grandfather Omo says so fondly, "normal as pie." A toddler who runs everywhere, chats about the most curiously obvious facts, and from time to time throws fits so grand that they make us laugh as extremely as they consume her. The PDA ligation that saved her life left her with a paralyzed left vocal fold. Although her first year was spent in silence—no cries, no screams—at around twelve months we heard her first, glorious chirps, and now she sometimes screams with no mercy at the grocery store where others stare and I knowingly chuckle. She has difficulty swallowing, for which we get twice weekly feeding therapy, and she is only able to consume liquids as thick as milkshakes. But this aside, if you didn't know her story, you wouldn't imagine it for her. You would not fathom what she has lived through.

And yet, pull back her shirt, put her in a tank top, watch her running in the yard through the sprinkler or splashing in the bath, and you will see that she wears her story on her skin. She seems to know the skin on her chest is different. Sometimes when she's only in a diaper, she grasps this thin skin between her thumbs and forefingers, pulling it away from her body and toward her father and me, showing it excitedly as if she is holding out a t-shirt whose message she wants us to read. And although our instincts now are to stop her so that she doesn't cause further injury, I wish for her that this could be how she always feels.

When she stands before a mirror some day, taking a closer look, I hope she regards the reflection of how her body worked, moment by moment, cell by cell, to repair the nearly mortal danger of her precarious circumstances. I hope that beneath the surface of her skin, she can feel her heart pounding with a mighty strength, the strength of two babies, both for herself who lives on and for her lost twin brother whose heart beats in hers.

Each night, after her bath, we rub her chest gently with cream, just like the dermatologist suggested during the consult. For this ritual, we have chosen a face cream rather than a body cream, whose extra richness we hope will give her the greatest possible benefit. I imagine that in some small way, this act gives her thanks, celebrates her as a victor, celebrates the vastness of our love for this mighty child and for the massive feats she has already achieved in her short life. And as I rub, I hope that someday when she tells the story of her skin, and perhaps notes that it is not the same as that of others, she recognizes just how beautiful that difference is.

I think back to a most tender baby shower prior to her release from the NICU. This, I remember thinking at the time, is a baby story I can understand. This is how it is supposed to be. But there was recognition at that party by a friend who had adopted, another who had lost a baby, a third who was a surrogate mother to so many on a university campus, and another still waiting to see if pregnancy was a possibility, that babies come to us in all sorts of ways, and sometimes not at all. I felt genuine happiness that day, that Isabel and I and our family were surrounded by the very best kind of love—an honest love. It seemed that no baby had ever been so celebrated, and the gifts were abundant. Gifts, held in cute sacks, stuffed with pastel rainbows of tissue paper. I peeled back the tissue to see what was inside. The best kind of surprise. The one that I couldn't have chosen better myself. The one that was just right.

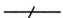

Perhaps both of our bodies have always belonged to medicine, its hard science and its magic, its tools that have opened us up and sealed us back, its actors who have chosen poorly or waited patiently or saved our lives. Neither of us will ever know what it feels like to live without scar tissue, to *not* have it mark us and guide us and guide the way that others interact with us. We were born with scars, we were born of scars. Because of our scars, we live. Despite all my surgeries and all of hers, there is no guarantee that we will not have more. In fact, for Isabel, a nerve reinervation surgery is on the horizon. It would sever the nerve that runs to her left vocal fold which was paralyzed by her PDA ligation and rejoin the fold with a functional nerve elsewhere in her neck with the ideal that it would enable close to normal swallowing function. It would attempt to resolve an early cut with a later cut. In terms of storytelling, a revision.

Our scars will continue to articulate, reticulate. Our skin will be filled up with all kinds of stories, and then revised, cut, rewritten. The story I have written of Isabel's scars is one I cannot separate from the ways that our family has scarred and healed along with her. The story I have written of her skin notes how something as gossamer and tenuous as tissue paper has held all of our lives together. I suppose in the end, the tissue was just as thick and sturdy as it needed to be.

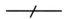

Narrative Adhesion

Shireen Campbell

Wounds heal,
Leave behind faint lines.
All admire, I admire,
The wound's wholeness healed,
The spirited recovery.

The tale of injury becomes currency
to circulate
at relevant programs and in select
office hour moments.

A narrative acolyte, I testify.
Telling our stories reclaims
the self. Reframes
the self.

Thickening syllables, narrative adhesion,
Tissued in words I have chosen.
Unsaid, unseen.
Faint pink in the light,
Deep red in the darkness.

—⫻—

WHY I (CAN'T) WRITE ABOUT SCARS

Gretchen Case

I.

The radiation treatment my mother underwent for non-Hodgkin's lymphoma required her to wear a mask of plastic mesh, molded precisely to her face, which held her head in position so that the radiation could be focused as narrowly as possible on the affected lymph nodes in her neck. After many weeks of use, her treatments were completed, and I asked her if I could keep the mask. On the inside, the contours of my mother's face were marked by remnants of her makeup: blush on cheeks, mascara on eyes, lipstick on mouth. The tools of cancer treatment had marked my mother, but she had marked those tools as well.

That re-creation of her face in featureless mesh was meant to immobilize her and isolate her unhealthy parts, and yet it provided evidence that she was vibrating with life inside. Earrings and a little bit of makeup were de rigueur before leaving the house. As my mother had explained to me many times throughout my adolescence, these were small signs that one had made an effort and thus a sign of respect to everyone encountered. In these smudges and smears, I saw a woman who was conducting business as usual, cancer be damned.

My mother died more than ten years ago, but I still have her mask. I also have the catheter that ran into the chemotherapy port in her chest, which—everyone tells me—is a gross thing to keep. But it was the scar from her port that first got me thinking about the ways in which medicine marks the body. I have more typical mementos, too—photos, videos, items of clothing. Once I understood that my mother might die, I felt a desperate need to gather evidence that she lived.

I also needed to make something important and useful out of my experience with her illness. The scar from her port and her radiation mask inspired an academic project that would investigate the ways that people respond to the marks left on them by medical interventions. This project became my doctoral dissertation, and led me to interview dozens of people about their scar stories. I studied the biological mechanisms of scar tissue and investigated the decisions of surgeons and physicians when placing, making, and closing incisions. I also researched risk factors for problems with scarring and potential treatments. I tried to become an expert on scars; in particular, I sought expertise in what scars mean to the people who bear them.

II.

We thought the little chirps coming from our one-day-old daughter were adorable; our nurse did not. Our little bundle was whisked down the hall to the Newborn Intensive Care Unit (NICU) for further evaluation. When I was finally allowed to see her again, she was ensconced in a padded plastic bassinet, intravenous lines running into her scalp, oxygen cannula in her nose, and heart monitor electrodes on her chest. Pneumonia, I was told. She'd have to stay in the NICU for at least a week.

Although I could barely walk after a complicated Caesarean delivery (which led to her pneumonia), my first thought was that I should grab her and run. I work in that hospital, and I knew the floor plan well enough that I figured I could get out before they caught us. Anything seemed better than the barbaric treatment she was getting. Such a tiny girl being poked and bled and filled with drugs.

Of course, I stayed. I could barely walk, let alone run away with her. I cried, but otherwise controlled my terror and consented to her treatment. I went out to the lobby to tell my husband, who was suffering from a cold and couldn't go anywhere near the fragile babies in the NICU. It would be days before he could see her again.

For the next few days, I stayed in a room on the other side of the building, recovering from multiple medical issues of my own. Every three hours, around the clock, I went to nurse my child, crossing through a busy corridor filled with my colleagues. Not even once was I recognized. In my robe and slippers, I blended into the patient population. On one of these visits to the NICU, the attending physician and the nurse wanted to talk to me about my baby's left arm. They showed me a large blister near her wrist and an open sore inside her elbow and explained that the placement of a new IV had not gone smoothly. I felt that feral anger rise up again and I was terse when I said that these wounds had better heal without scarring.

As a scholar, I had argued that each scar must have unique meaning for its bearer and that those individual stories must be affected by cultural narratives. Scars provide evidence of a body interacting with the world. They can be part of a conqueror's narrative, connoting bravery, strength, perseverance. They can be part of a martyr's narrative, connoting damage, weakness, vulnerability. And they can be part of a criminal's narrative, connoting danger, violence, ugliness. In my dissertation, I rejected the idea of scar as pure metaphor because that ignores the physical realities of living with scar tissue.

Despite all this work, I'm not sure I ever went beyond my own, selective meaning-making. The scholar in me hoped to understand scars in a new and productive way but the mother in me saw only damage to my child. I struggled between intellectual appraisal of the scars and maternal rage. I knew good and well that scarring is unpredictable, that her doctors had not intentionally harmed or neglected her, and that sometimes even simple medical procedures have complications. Yet I kept badgering them. I wanted them to feel terrible about ruining my baby's perfect skin.

Her elbow healed, but her wrist still carries a small, bubble-shaped, raised scar, barely noticeable to anyone but me. But to me, that scar says that I could have lost her in any of a million unpredictable ways and that I still could, that our human bodies are fragile. And yet I had argued that I didn't want scars to be symbols.

III.

A tiny cyst, just an annoyance near the nape of my neck. I wanted it gone. Itchy? Sure. Painful? OK. Affecting my quality of life? Um, yes. I wanted it gone, and I was agreeable to any suggested description that would make it go away faster.

The surgery itself was barely surgery. A little something injected to numb the area. Some pressure and then a painful *pop* and an exclamation from the physician: "Oh! That was deeper than it looked." I didn't say anything, but I was surprised at her surprise. I marked that moment, in the way that you mark slightly unusual moments that may or may not turn out later to be of significance.

As the incision healed, it did not smooth out and I developed a keloid. The reasons that some people develop these puffy, painful scars are not entirely clear, although there are some recognized risk factors. I don't fit into the usual demographic of younger, darker skin, although my keloid is located in what this dermatologist called the "Bermuda Triangle" of the upper back, neck and shoulders.

I returned twice to the same dermatologist for steroid injections to flatten the scar but there was not much change. I had to decide whether to try more aggressive treatments or to live with the lump that was larger and more troublesome than the original cyst. The shiny, pale skin of the keloid was quite visible against my freckles and constantly bothered me as it rubbed against collars, necklaces, and purse straps. The vanity that this scar revealed bothered me more than anything else. The keloid, relatively small, changed the way I dressed and moved. I turned my collars up and wore my hair down. Where was the courage and acceptance of scars that I celebrated in other people?

I am at peace with the many surgical scars across my abdomen, which are easily covered by clothing. Because I can control who sees those scars, I can control who knows their stories. This keloid, though, misbehaved in plain sight. If I were truly an expert on scars, if I believed my own arguments, I would celebrate this keloid's narrative power, right? Instead, I resented it. I made an appointment with a different dermatologist.

He looked at the lump carefully and gave me a number of options for treatment. With his guidance, I chose to try a higher dose of injected steroids to see if it would reduce the size and relieve the itching and burning. I left his office with instructions to massage the area several times a day to help distribute the drug evenly. Over the next week, I fell into the habit of keeping my hand on my neck, constantly manipulating the scar. I was sitting at a friend's house about ten days after that injection, rubbing my neck absentmindedly, when it burst. Like, really *burst*. Luckily, my friend was not rattled by this scene from a horror movie. My sense of liberation when the lump burst was twofold. The relief of pain and itching was almost instantaneous. Less welcome was my guilty pleasure at feeling the lump become a deep indentation and knowing at once that this was not a keloid. Which meant that it might go (mostly) away.

A return trip to the second dermatologist confirmed that original cyst had not been completely removed. Multiple steroid injections shrunk the surrounding healthy tissue, allowing the cyst to grow quickly larger until it became the shiny lump on my neck. Now his challenge was to figure out how to repair the divot left behind; surgery was scheduled. I chatted with him through the whole procedure, learning new colloquialisms like "tram tracks" (the dots alongside a main scar that I've always thought of as "Frankenstein stitches") and "step-offs" (when the skin doesn't come together properly and heals on an uneven plane). Although it was minor surgery, once again there were surprises in the way my skin and tissue behaved. The surgery lengthened, and so did the scar, to about three inches.

This new scar is healing nicely, but it is much more noticeable than the cyst or the faux-keloid. Nobody ever commented on those, in part because they were smaller and in part because I kept them hidden. Now, however, I frequently hear that question asked so often of the people I interviewed for my dissertation: "What happened?!" One of my physician colleagues walking behind me down the hallway intoned, "I see the mark of man upon you."

But here's the thing: this scar looks like a scar. It is a long, thin, shiny, pinkish-white line with a few smaller lines branching off. The surgeon made sure that the scar neatly followed the natural lines of cleavage on my neck, and that the edges came together tightly. It's a textbook scar, already fading into the surrounding terrain, just as it is supposed to do. This scar behaves. And I have a pretty good scar story, not terribly dramatic, but still one that resonates with anyone who has had a small physical irritation turn into a medical saga, consuming time and money.

IV.

When I researched and wrote my dissertation, I think what I wanted was for scars to be discrete prompts for stories that provide explanations. Maybe I chose the topic because a specific set of scar stories—my mother's—were unsatisfactory. They didn't yield a narrative that explained why she would get sick and die. When confronted with scars on the body of my child, I did not want any narratives at all, except one that would end with no scars. This followed the story told in medical texts proclaiming that the ideal scar is the invisible scar, a standard that I had roundly criticized and nevertheless embraced in the NICU. And when confronted with a visible, but truly minor, scar of my own, I showed none of the resilience and imagination I had celebrated in my interviewees. Instead, I complained and persisted until I got a scar that looked like what I thought a scar should look like.

My attempts to report on the meanings others make of their scars sound hollow to me now. In hollow spaces, echoes thrive; my voice, repeating endlessly what I want scars to mean for others, what I hope scars will not mean for me. Every scar generates multiple narratives that upset histories as both scars and stories shift and change. Scars not only have meaning, they make meaning. I recognize the powerful ways that many people use the stories of their scars to shape their experience in the world. I also recognize the powerful social narratives that work against individual meaning-making. The desire for smooth skin with only minimal, recognizable flaws easily overwhelmed my scholarly understanding of productive difference. I'm still searching for an honest way to write about scars, one that acknowledges my reverence for scars on other bodies but not on my own. The terms of that hypocritical stance, I think, might be something really worth studying.

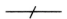

REMOVAL

Natalie Karneef

Come close and you probably still won't see it. It's a tiny circle, barely etched in my skin. More of an emptiness than an actual scar.

But I see it. Or rather, I feel it—the absence it leaves. I run my hand over it: its smoothness, its cleanness, the space it left behind. And I feel in control. Not of everything, but of what counts.

I was twenty-seven when I made the decision, but I can't recall why. Was it simply that I passed a dermatologist's office every day on my way to the metro station, and so was prompted, at about 8:30 each morning, to consider removing this thing that had been with me all my life? Or did I need another one taken off, perhaps one that was unsightly or suspicious? Did I ask, offhand, if the doctor could get rid of this one, too, like a two-for-one deal? I no longer recall.

This sounds so dramatic.

Truth? I'm talking about a mole. Not a cancerous one. Not a dangerous-looking one, even, as much as I tried to convince doctors otherwise. You could even call it a beauty mark, but I never did. To me, it was ugly, protruding, intrusive. Most importantly, my mother had the exact same one, in the exact same spot–just to the right of the navel, and a little bit north.

I was shocked at how easy it was to get rid of. A shot of anesthetic, the swipe of a scalpel, and voilà. It was like it had never existed. The doctor charged me $10 on top of the Medicare bill, because it was for cosmetic reasons, but I probably would've handed over $1,000, if I'd had it.

I watched him stick the bloody remains in a jar. He said, "Just to make sure all is okay." He meant, *Just to make sure it isn't cancer.* I thought, *Just to make sure she is gone.*

After the surgery, I would have a small indentation in my skin, and one less connection to my mother. That's how I viewed it, anyway. As I watched the doctor turn the jar lid, I considered the memories I would get surgically removed, if I could. I imagined him hermetically sealing the worst week of my childhood in that jar so that it would never be seen again.

———/———

I wish I could tell you that Simon was tall and muscly, or tattooed and shaved, or at least Doc Martened up the yin yang. Alas. Simon, white-t-shirt-white-sneakers-and-blue-jeans-Simon, was the kind of guy fathers of sixteen-year-old daughters pray for. Top of the class. Played the violin. Went to math camp, for godsakes. But he loved Led Zeppelin and building campfires, and was one of the kindest, gentlest males I'd ever met. Plus, he had a car. He was supposed to be tutoring me in biology that day, but instead, like all self-respecting teenagers, we went to the mall.

I wasn't allowed to hang out at the mall, especially not with boys. My immigrant parents didn't believe in either, nor did they believe in parties, dating, or contact lenses. Naturally, their iron-fisted rule created a first-class liar. I was "having dinner at my aunt's house" the first time I did acid; "sleeping at my best friend's house" when I experienced my first mosh pit. My father was away on business a lot around then, and my mom was getting worse, in direct proportion to his absence. Slapping me more often. Hiding my posters under rugs, my books in hallway closets. Coming into my room after I'd gone to bed, pulling me from my bed, ordering me to dust the baseboards or clean the kitchen sink.

I felt her before I saw her, that day at the mall. Simon and I were in front of the photo developing store, and I smelled her perfume, maybe, or recognized the sound of her steps from behind. Then her hand was around my arm, yanking hard, disgust dripping from her heavy Hungarian hiss, and I was aflame in humiliation as Simon, confused and helpless, watched her drag me out to the parking lot.

I'm sure there was a slap or two when we got home, if not before. That was standard. I was sent to my room in the basement, where I huddled in my closet in a ball of shame and tears until night fell. Who knows what I thought, or said to myself, or wrote. But after a while, hungry and spent from crying, I tiptoed upstairs, hoping to be allowed the amnesty of some ice cream and TV.

Within seconds of my ascent, there was the pounding of feet, the stabbing pain of my hair being pulled, the jolt of being pushed downstairs and onto the basement floor. The next part is a blur of elbows, of punches and kicks and screams, of curling up like an insect, pleading, wailing. The feeling of the carpet and the grey-blue color of the walls are imprinted in my mind. So is exactly where I was sitting, how close it was to the stairs, which led to the garage, which led to outside, and how far to freedom that distance felt. We lived on fifty acres in the middle of the country. The closest house was two kilometers away, and home to a pair of suntanned, tennis-playing parents and a girl my age who wore matching scrunchies and socks and led the cheerleading team. I had no driver's license, and there were no cell phones.

I don't recall the rest of that night. Who knows how I processed what had happened, or what I plotted. I just know that the next day—getting onto my school bus, passing the neighbours bouncing merrily into their SUV—felt like a great escape. I didn't know how I would avoid it, but I knew I wasn't going back home. And knowing that was fucking paradise.

I don't know what I told the first guidance counselor.

I remember being called out of class later on, the rattling fear in my chest, wondering if everyone could tell just by looking at me.

And I remember the meeting: me on one side of a desk, a jury of frowning adults on the other. Had this happened before? How often? What do you mean, every week? Once a week? More? Really? Does your father hit you? Are you sure? Does your mom ever try to touch you in bad places? Are you sure? More questions, more offices, a lot of scribbling on clipboards. It was surreal, like a dream, but at the same time, it felt, to my surprise, good. So good. Reassuring, like maybe I was right. Like maybe I didn't deserve this. Like maybe none of it had ever been okay.

I stayed at my best friend's house for the rest of the week, borrowing her boyfriend's oversized basketball fleece with sleeves that covered my hands, wishing I could stop time and feel this safe forever.

Later, after my dad got back from his trip, we all went to see the social worker together. Also—and this was the best part—I got to go see her alone. I bathed in the warmth of her concern, relished her questions, drank in her soft voice, mused over her table covered in miniature plastic animals. She confirmed that I had done the right thing; that no matter what I did, I didn't deserve to be hit. Too bad it took me many more years to believe her.

When I was in first year university, mother thanked me for speaking up. She said it was me who'd had the courage to point to the cracks that were appearing, who brought to light the fine lines which were now splintering into divorce and monumental legal battles. But she never talked about why it happened. When I brought it up, a few years ago, she said she didn't remember that week. Then she asked why I didn't blame my father for never being around.

You're hanging onto the past, she told me. *You need to let go. Anyway, it never happened again.*

Not with your fists, I replied.

She hung up the phone.

We didn't talk for two years.

———/———

But the 10-second surgery didn't slice my mother away.

Her constant judgment, her unending weigh-ins and unattainable standards: they're all still in there, alive and kicking. I work too hard and not hard enough. I spend too much money on health food and don't take good enough care of myself. I'm too thin and too chubby. I'm overdressed and look like a homeless person. I'm always late or so early that I didn't plan my day properly. I rush into things and can't make decisions.

Even after years of meditation and therapy, I sometimes forget that hers is just another voice that I don't have to believe.

But when I run my hand across my stomach, I feel the tiny circle of what once was there. Touching that emptiness, I am reminded that the more I pay attention, the more I will remember: her mark is gone. It never will exist again. And I was the one who got rid of it.

I took back what was mine.

The power I didn't know I had.

The possibility.

———/———

•

And We Closed Our Eyes

Lea Ervin

"Fuck you, you piece of shit."
I hurled the bloody metal nail file into the mirror.

Furiously, I glared at my own reflection while gripping the white counter top with my bloody hands. My breath was on fire. I was on fire. My body was fueled with adrenaline after stabbing myself with the file after my bath.

Why, you ask? *Because why the fuck not?* My body was attacking me, so I decided to give it a taste of its own vile medicine. That's what happens when you have an autoimmune disease. It renders you helpless, so you have to find a way to reclaim power.

Endometriosis took my power.

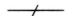

I was diagnosed after years of suffering with what I thought was "my normal." Apparently, crippling abdominal pain was "all in my head," and "my lot in life." Actually, these were bullshit clichés I was handed by doctor after doctor until I finally had my first diagnostic laparoscopy on June 13, 2009. This surgery left me with two small scars—nothing unsightly or major.

The surgery helped for about a year, but then the original symptoms, burning urination, constant abdominal cramping, and bowel incontinence, returned. My ObGyn was reluctant to operate a second time, but she did. This time, I was left with three more small scars to add to a growing collection. Afterward, she urged me to try hormone therapy. She gave me two options: Depo Provera or Lupron. My memory fails me as to what good the Depo Provera was supposed to do, but I remember clearly the words "will kill the endometriosis" with regard to Lupron.

"Kill it?" I asked?
"Yes."
"Well, let's do that one, then" was my obvious answer.
"It's an expensive injection, so we'll have to check with your insurance first to see if they'll cover it. But I doubt there will be an issue since it was proven by biopsy that you have endometriosis. Once we get approval, we'll call you back in to give you the injection," explained my doctor.

"Sounds good."

I went home and felt relieved, hoping for a cure. But of course, what seems to be "too good to be true" usually is. A friend of mine, who had taken Lupron shots for endometriosis, urged me to reconsider.

"Don't do it," she said.

"It'll ruin your life," she said.

"You'll regret it," she said.

I should have listened. Instead, I agreed to take my first of two injections over a six-month period.

First, my hair fell out. When I brushed my hair at night, clumps would form in the brush. Bald spots began to appear like small islands in a sea of black. I lost twenty pounds from my one hundred ten pound frame, my breasts swelled to a ridiculous size and ached every day, and I lost my shit. I went crazy.

My blood boiled twenty-four hours a day, which left me with a need to attack whatever was in my path. My husband, friends, and family never knew who they would encounter on a given day—Mrs. Hyde or Mrs. Jekyll. Mrs. Hyde appeared most frequently. My friends were reluctant to spend any time with me for fear of having their heads ripped off; my parents cringed when the phone rang and played a nightly game of "paper, rock, scissors" to determine the poor soul plagued with the task of taking my call. The irony is "mood swings" were listed under Lupron's "less serious side effects," even though they did the most damage.

My husband, Brock, was married to a maniac corpse of a woman who hated him. We had only been married for two years, and already our marriage was circling the drain. We fought daily over nothing. He never wanted to come home. Why would he? Home was a nightmare.

I was aware of how everyone felt about me, yet I couldn't stop myself when my eyes started to burn with anger, my mouth would twist with fury, my skin would tingle with vitriol, and I would erupt. My attacks were mostly verbal, but at times, would become physical. When Brock was on the receiving end, he would patiently take it without any retaliation. Until one night, on our back porch, he became fed up.

"So who is she?" The words slithered out of my mouth and crawled their way into his ears. I crossed my legs arrogantly and flicked the ashes from my cigarette. I blew the smoke in his direction as I rocked back and forth in the metal bench swing.

"Who is who?" he asked, annoyed. "What are you talking about?"

"Whoever it is you're fucking." I snarled back.

Since the injections, I'd had terrible bouts of paranoia along with anger. Brock never gave me a reason to believe he was cheating on me; however, his cheating was my biggest fear. Somehow, this drug "treatment" coaxed me into entertaining my nightmares. These thoughts were enticing. They wanted me to play with them and indulge them. So, I did.

"I'm not doing this," he answered blankly.

"Ha, why not? I'm just curious *what* is it about her? Is she taller? Skinnier? Bigger tits? What? Which is it?" I asked as the volume of my voice increased with each question until it erupted into a scream. "*Which is it!?*" I hurtled a beer bottle at him. He leaped out of the way and the bottle crashed into the wall.

"You know what? This is bullshit. You are sick—like mentally fucked up. You're a horrible person. I'm done here. I think everyone is done with you. I'm the last one you had on your side, and I'm fucking finished. I'd rather be alone for the rest of my life than live with you one more minute." He was shuddering with rage.

He walked out back in the house and left me fuming on the bench swing. I gathered myself. Stubbed the cigarette out in the ashtray, and sauntered back in. "Fuck you," I said blankly as I passed him on my way to the bathroom. He looked right through me and didn't respond. I drew a bath, took off my clothes, and looked in the mirror.

"Ugh. Gross," fell from my lips.

The water warmly received my right foot, then my left foot, my buttocks, my back, and then my stomach. The water ebbed and flowed over my belly, washing over my surgical scars, and receded. What if the water could cleanse my body of this illness and erase the scars? What if it were that easy? What if I could step out of this tub as if it were a baptismal font and I could be new? Clean? Forgiven? If only. As I stepped out of the tub, I began to replay our fight and I heard the first sob escape my mouth. Another followed until I was choking on them. When I grew tired of the water, the towel embracing me was the only comfort available as I had alienated everything else. The mirror was my foe. There were no barriers left—no makeup, no hairstyles, no clothes. Everything in front of me was the truth—the failing body that wasn't healthy enough, pretty enough. My body was simply not enough.

So I snatched the nearest sharp object I could find. With the metal nail file, I began to stab. I cut my breasts. I went for them first because they weren't big enough to keep my husband from other women. I cut my thighs since they were fat and cellulite ridden. They were already gross. Why not make them worse? And then my abdomen. It housed my uterus. That piece of shit was trying to kill me. The agony it caused me was brutal. I lived with the pain of what felt like a thousand white hot knives penetrating my naval, vagina, and rectum. This Lupron was supposed to kill it, wasn't it? Isn't that what the doctor promised? Lies! I stabbed and stabbed until I exhausted myself. Then I slammed the nail file into the mirror, clutched the counter top, and collapsed on to the floor.

"*What the hell are you doing?*" Brock screamed as he burst through the bathroom door and found me. He wrapped himself around me and restrained my arms so I wouldn't harm myself further and lifted me to my feet.

"*Why did you do this? Why!? What the hell is wrong with you?*" he screamed as I bucked and tried to fight him off. I couldn't though. He was too big—too powerful. He was full of life, and I was not.

"I wanted to," I stammered. What else was I supposed to do? Everyone hates me. I hate myself."

"*Goddammit, Lea! Goddammit!*" He clutched my shoulders and shook me, pulling me into himself in an embrace. "What are you doing, baby? We gotta do something. We gotta do something," he sobbed as he rocked me from side to side.

"Do what?" I whimpered. "What's left?"

Brock and I spent the entire night grasping at straws, trying to come up with a solution. We first decided that regardless of what any physician said, I would not take the second injection. Next, we agreed on getting a second opinion. For all we knew, there could've been a much easier approach to treating endometriosis. Last, we promised never to give up on each other.

"How are we going to make it through this? I asked him.

"Well, we'll just close our eyes and duck."

And, we did. We visited my new doctor. She gave me three options: Lupron again, another laparoscopy, or a total hysterectomy.

"I'll give you two time to talk," she said as she left the room to write me a prescription for pain medicine. Brock and I looked at each other for a few minutes.

"Well Lupron is out," I said.

"So, all that's left is surgery. The last laps didn't work. If you're going to do surgery again, I think we should be done," Brock answered.

Done meaning the hysterectomy. He was right, though. Nothing else had worked, and this was our last option. The thought of such a surgery was horrifying; however, that horror was also a beacon of hope.

"Let's be done, then."

We waited in silence.

As we waited, I replayed the night after the bath in my head. That would be my life if I didn't have the hysterectomy. That person in the bathroom wasn't me; it was some monster. I needed to get back to being me again.

We heard the creak of the door and in walked the doctor.

"So, what are we going to do?" she asked.

"We . . . we're . . . I'm . . . going to have a hysterectomy." I thought of children. My children. The children I would never have.

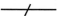

I signed my name and wrote the date: July 25, 2011. I handed the pen and clipboard back to my doctor and looked at her for a moment, examining her expression. Was everyone judging me for my decision? The hospital bed was cold and hard as I slumped back with a sigh and waited for the pre-op nurse to start the IV. As I waited, my eyes scanned the room, settling on the curtains that separated me from the other patients. Ugly fabric. Faded orange, sprinkled with green and blue squares.

"Who thought this design was a good idea?" I mumbled to myself in my usual snarky tone.

It was freezing. The hospital gown only made me feel more vulnerable, and it dressed me in more ugly fabric. The only things that helped were the light blue, hospital-issued socks. I pulled them up to my knees and tried my hardest to cozy up under the stiff sheet and rough blanket.

"*What will become of me? Sixteen years of suffering with endometriosis is enough, right?*"

I heard the swish of the curtain, and in walked a thin nurse in blue scrubs, her red hair clipped back in a chignon. A few rogue strands fell in front of her green eyes. She had a delicate face with alabaster skin on the cusp of aging, but not quite there yet. She smiled. I returned a smile.

In a soft Irish accent, she informed me, "I'm going to hook up your IV now. First, I need you to look over this and make sure it's all correct."

I took the clipboard from her and examined the paperwork. My name, age, address, and procedure were all there. All correct. I handed her the clipboard and offered my left hand. She tied off my arm with the rubber strap. It squeezed against my skin like the Indian sunburn my friends and I used to give each other as children. Then came the numbness and tingle. I felt the cold swab of alcohol wisp across my hand which she quickly fanned so it would evaporate a little. Then the pop of the safety cap from the needle. She found a vein on the first stick. My thick, dark blood snaked its way up the tube. The rush of the cold saline filled my hand and crept up into my arm. She hooked a bag of what I assume was antibiotics on the IV pole and turned on the compression machine that was attached to my legs. It began to contract.

Squeeze.

Release.

Squeeze.

Release.

"I'll go get your family now," she said gently.

"Please," I replied. She left and there I sat for my last few minutes alone. I didn't have my iPod with me so I had no music, but "Try, Try, Try" by The Smashing Pumpkins played in my head—a song I had loved for many years.

"Try to hold on . . . a little bit longer. Try to hold on . . ." I hummed to myself. I was holding on, Billy. I was doing my best.

"Hey, love." It was Brock, followed by my Mom and Dad. They filed in and, one by one, gave me kisses and hugs. I had my entire family's support which was nice, but I was unsure if I had my own support.

"How do you feel?" asked my mom.

"Fine. Nervous."

"You'll be alright," she said in her usual, reassuring tone.

The nurse quickly came back in and began to inject something into my IV. She fumbled with some cords and uncapped the syringe and injected some medication that burned a bit at first, but then a wave of softness enveloped me. I melted into the bed.

"It's Versed. It'll help you relax a bit, yeah?" she said with a laugh. "I can see it's already working." It was working. After a bit of slurred conversation and a few laughs at my expense, the OR nurse came in to discuss my surgery.

"Hello Elizabeth, what's your birthday? "

"July 31, 1982."

"Oh you have a birthday in a few days. Happy early birthday."

"Thanks?"

Happy flippin' birthday to me. Everyone wants to turn twenty-nine while recovering from the major abdominal surgery which took away all reproductive organs.

"Can you tell me what procedure you'll be having this morning?" she asked blankly. It was apparent she asked this question many times a day.

"Total hysterectomy. Tubes, ovaries . . . everything," I answered in the same blank manner.

"You do understand that after this surgery, you will no longer be able to have children," she insisted.

"Yes. I signed the form when I got here."

"Okay then, I'll give you a minute with your family."

I hugged them all again. Brock kissed my forehead as he'd done many times, before many surgeries. The patient care tech released the breaks of my gurney which jolted me out of my euphoria. It was about to happen. I looked at my family. For a split second, I went over the decision in my head again. *Is the right thing? I'm letting my family down. I have no children and will never have children. I'm cheating everyone I love. I'm choosing to castrate myself all because I live in pain. I can tough it out for a while longer, right?*

"Wait!" I cried as I sat up with a start. "Wait, just give me a minute." I looked back a Brock. I looked into his blue eyes for what seemed like an eternity. He nodded. He smiled. He said, "We'll be okay, love." I looked at my mother. I saw the potential in her to be a wonderful grandmother just like my Meme was to me. I looked at my father. I saw the opportunity to teach his grandson how to throw a football slip away from him all because of me. *How could I do this to them? I was an only child, their only chance.* But then my dad smiled and said, "We'll see you on the other side." That was all I needed.

"Okay, let's do this then," I stammered.

My last memories of that day were the rush of the cold when we entered the operating room, and the icy feel of the operating table. They said the surgery went well. I woke up feeling a dull pain in my abdomen. It wasn't the usual burning sharpness of the endometriosis pain. In the coming months, I would learn what it would be like to live without chronic, debilitating pain. And in that moment, I felt some relief.

I wish I could say life was perfect after, but real life isn't. Adjusting to being menopausal at twenty-nine years old was quite a challenge. Hot flashes, migraines, and insomnia were new challenges I had to overcome, but at least they weren't endometriosis. At least they weren't Lupron.

Many people couldn't quite grasp why I would choose such an extreme. "How could you do this to yourself?" "How could you do this to Brock? He'd be such a good dad." "How could you give up the joy of children?" "You must be a selfish person, then." Baby shower invitations stopped coming. Friends were weird about telling me they were pregnant. I was hurt by the fact others thought I had given up sharing their joy and given up joy, period.

I took my joy back. I had to sacrifice some, but I took it back.

I have ten scars total. They scatter over a once smooth stomach like little fault lines. Remnants of unrest. I am not embarrassed by them. To me, they represent everything that I tolerated, fought through, and won. My mother calls them "my badges of honor." That's a little hokey, but she's right. They are a part of who I am now at age thirty-two. They remind me, that no matter what, I will survive.

As far as the experience with Lupron, I wish I could say I've moved on. It scarred me more than a scalpel ever could. We all have darkness inside of us; however, most people never let it surface. I came face-to-face with my worst self in the mirror that night in the bathroom. I wish I could spout off the, "I've learned from it and have become a better person because of it" blather like I'm supposed to, but looking back, I feel nothing but regret for the way I treated myself and my loved ones. Becoming aware of my darkness was the most frightening part of the experience. I'm afraid "Lupron Lea" will make an appearance again in the future, and this time, there will be no forgiveness.

One evening, after reflecting on this illness, I asked Brock, "How did we do it? How did we make it?

"Well, I guess we just closed our eyes and ducked," he answered with a laugh.

He was right. We just closed our eyes. It was all we could do.

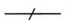

Mending with Gold

Jennifer Stager

On the night that Peter fell, his blood covered me. Less than you'd guess given how close to death he lay with his unmoving eyes jerked up to the right, but enough that I washed up my forearms and changed my clothes before putting the children to bed. Enough that a friend came by later to mop the cracked pavement outside of our house, to which Peter had fallen from the landing of our apartment a story up. He'd been helping a friend move a bureau, lost his footing on a shoddy stair repair, and fallen over the side of the stairwell.

I was still slapping his face and shouting his name when a neighbor ran across the street, already calling 911. In those long minutes on the line, I debated whether to run the short distance to the hospital, but finally I heard the sirens starting up from the hospital lot. The paramedics arrived and took over; one of them ushered me aside and gestured toward the apartment where our children's three faces were pressed to the bay window.

"It is going to be a while before you can see him, so I suggest you put the children to bed before you come down. The hospital will be a crazy place for them."

This made sense, but I feared leaving Peter alone, accompanied only by paramedics and the machines that had already taken over for his failing body. I ran to the open back of the ambulance for one last "I love you!" before they drove the few blocks down the hill. All of those months of hearing sirens rush past our house to or from the hospital and tonight the sirens shrilled for us.

Perhaps fifteen minutes had passed since Peter had come home from work, greeted our neighbors, and said, "Let's get this done," before taking the heavy end of the bureau we were giving away. It was not surprising that he chose the downhill position where the angle pushed much of the bureau's weight onto him; he has always been the person to shoulder the heavier load.

——/——

Inside our apartment, I shifted into action, called my brother and my best friend, went to the bathroom to wash. I left his blood on my upper arm, where it streaked across my freckled birth mark, the one that my brother shares. In that shallowly breathing part of my mind, I thought it better to keep some of Peter's life force out of the drain and on my own living body.

Somehow I got our children to bed. I sang, and nursed, and rocked, and imagined so many scenarios of possible futures in fast little frames. My mind kept flashing forward, but I didn't land anywhere for long. If you know a song well, you can sing it without even hearing yourself, your mind fully absorbed by other thoughts, your person split.

My brother arrived, as did my friend. The baby fell asleep and I leaned over the guardrail to place her in the crib. I stopped singing. My brother walked me the few blocks to the large public hospital with the only Level One trauma center in San Francisco, where all the car accident and gun shot victims are treated. Peter would have ended up here eventually no matter where his accident had occurred, so our proximity was our first blessing. Perhaps ten minutes elapsed between the impact of his body on the concrete and the paramedics' arrival.

In the weeks that followed, I was grateful for the short walk that let me come and go between the hospital world and our children's lives throughout the day. My final visit of the day was always after dark, while a rotation of friends watched over our sleeping children from our living room couch. As I walked along the overpass, I watched the lighted cars moving along the freeway below, sparks of so many different lives. That first night I had lacked the ability to see the lighted cars and imagine other's distant lives some breaking apart, others mending. I had only been able to concentrate on breathing.

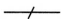

"It is like a window" the neurosurgeon explained after he had successfully operated on Peter's brain. "We open the skull plate, remove the expanding blood that is putting pressure on the brain, and then shut it again."

Dark, horizontal staples, each traced in dried blood, sutured the seam of his flesh and kept that window closed. Over time, Peter's skin would absorb the staples themselves, leaving only their small white marks in neat rows running parallel to his incision. I recognized this healing process from my own scar across my lower abdomen, where staples had held closed the opening from which my daughter had been pulled, feet first, little more than a year before Peter's fall.

"To the knee, the hip, the shoulder, and out," the doctor had narrated her birth, so different from the pressure and burning that had accompanied her brothers' head-first entrances into the world. Minutes later, as I struggled not to pass out from the anesthesia, a resident and a medical student discussed the virtues of staples versus stitches while they closed this gap in my flesh with immaculate precision. Babies who emerge from the birth canal can tear flesh as well, less evenly than a scalpel. A midwife had stitched those wounds with thread that my body had absorbed, leaving deeply hidden marks of mended and remended flesh.

Window. I pictured this analogy so often in the days that become weeks following Peter's surgery when he remained in the trauma ICU. The operation itself was the most straight-forwardly successful piece of his recovery. Twelve hours after he'd fallen to the concrete from the second story, a surgeon had successfully opened a window into his head, removed the blood pooling outside of the dura, the net, that holds his brain, and relieved what would have quickly become fatal pressure. Twelve days after those twelve hours, doctors successfully removed the ventilator that had taken over for his weakening rattle at the scene.

It would be several weeks more in the strobe-light mania of the ICU before Peter himself yanked out the drain that monitored the levels of his cerebral spinal fluid. "It looks like pee," my younger son said as, during an exceptional visit, he pointed to the clear bag suspended next to his father's head into which drained the liquid building up around his brain. That was the first permission I had given in the immediate aftermath of his accident, permission to drill through Peter's skull to place the monitor—a thin filament—inside his head.

How he reached his head with both hands tied to the hospital bed, none of us can figure. A nurse practitioner assured me that typical laws of physics do not bind patients with injured brains. The stories about other brain injuries that people shared with me often included moments of mania in the ICU—the concert producer remembered nothing of trying to strike his nurses, nor the Texan of leaping up from his bed shortly after the surgeon had removed all that he could of the tumor. One night Peter insisted that the curtain separating his bed from the other patient's bed concealed a shower, not a frail, elderly man on a ventilator. Peter had been bedridden for weeks and had yet to begin the painstaking work of relearning to walk, but he put up a good fight trying to get to that shower until his nurse signaled to the orderlies. Many patients do not realize that they cannot extricate their hands from the wrist ties and padded boxing gloves, cannot crunch forward on the bed and tear some tube from their head or nose or urethra. Not knowing that these movements should be impossible, they do find some way to escape, at least until the next round of sedation.

By New Year's Day, Peter had stabilized enough that I asked his nurse to help me shave his entire head. New year, new scalp. I managed the left side on my own, but had to ask her to shave around the incision itself, now firmly closed but still raw. Seven weeks of residential rehabilitation followed, during which time his curly, salty black hair slowly began to grow around the scar. His colleagues threw a fundraiser for him, at which many of them shaved their heads to match. By this time Peter's hair had grown in, so a hairdresser friend brought her supplies to the brain injury center and buzzed his hair, adding in patterns that riffed off of the arc of his scar, wending the long red arc into larger patterns of swirls and straight-edges. Between the hair and the Carhartts, he was officially the biggest hipster in rehab.

As the weeks blended into months, I found I inadvertently collected stories of other people's injured brains—the friend of a friend who'd been severely beaten on his way home from a ball game, the young Texan with the glamorous wife who'd been airlifted from Tahoe with a massive tumor, the newlywed art director in the car accident, the younger man whose off-road vehicle had flipped, leaving a horseshoe-shaped scar running the entire front of his scalp, the middle-aged man who'd been biking alone on Mt. Tam, the producer who fell thirty-five feet from the stage he was building for a rock star, the beautiful son who drove a motorcycle too young and now might never walk. These changed lives now intersected briefly with ours and I added them to my cup of stories.

At the start of Peter's hospitalization I took to drinking my morning tea out of a mug from the first major company that Peter worked for as a teenager. This dot-com had been a poster child for the excesses of the late 90s and many of Peter's friends had worked there in some capacity. Somehow, despite the stock plunging everyone out of a job, that mug had survived our many moves. "We handle the world's email," read the letters along the inside of the rim. Drinking from this particular mug became something of a ritual, one that in moments of utter uncertainty, I feared to break. Hospital days became weeks and Peter did not move. One morning I splashed hot water over the rim and dropped the mug in surprise. The handle broke off completely, leaving only sharp stumps.

A Japanese technique from the fifteenth century, *kintsugi*, mends pottery with gold. The glimmering lines mark the joins between fragments, highlighting rather than masking breaks and subsequent repairs. So beautiful appeared the mended vessels that some apparently took to smashing their unblemished cups, necessitating a repair in gold, a material long valued for its capacity to resist debasement. Air and water do not tarnish gold and the lustrous material can be shaped to fill gaps and join fragments. Kintsugi foregrounds the story of a damaged vessel's survival. If I brought the pieces of Peter's mug to a golden joiner, he could re-attach the handle to its body, leaving an exquisite line of gold to mark its moment of damage. For now, I simply hold the hot body to drink my tea, the sharp breaks at the handle rotated away from my lips.

After three months in three different hospitals, Peter came home. Although we'd had hints during the carefully staged hospital visits that rejoining our family of five would prove the greatest and most enduring trial, nothing had prepared us for this reality. A carefully repaired person had replaced the robust man who'd left us so suddenly. Fissures in the children emerged almost immediately, having been only shored up during those fugue months with a temporary gum.

"You left us! You went away and I had to *be* Papa!" shouted my oldest son one morning a few weeks after Peter had come home. All Peter could register in that moment was the shouting, not the words of someone not-yet seven, not the words of a child who could not make sense of everything he had seen. His younger brother spoke with little fists followed by gasping wails.

"We want the old Papa back!" they often cried. They searched widely for someone to blame for the accident—me, Papa, our uninjured friend, the landlords and their penny-pinching repairs, and finally, themselves. One night I navigated between our middle child screaming that I had wanted Papa to fall and that is why I had offered our friends the bureau, and our oldest crying that he did not deserve to be loved, that he wished he were dead. "I wish," he gasped, "that my sperm had never met the egg." Eventually his sobs subsided into sleep.

The baby, who had barely spoken at the time of the accident, now knew the word "cane" and kept a close eye on her father's. "Papa fall," she would announce seemingly out of nowhere and at first I did not hear the underlying question. Over time I learned to respond with a bright, "but now he is ok," as though assuring her could make it so.

The children had mistaken the hospital stay for a way-station from which their old papa would eventually return. All those months of tardy slips, gifted casseroles, missed homework, and rotating nighttime sitters, had, they hoped, just been part of this waiting place. They could not see much gold in the taciturn, jerking man who took their father's place, with his misshapen words, halting steps, and need for endless quiet.

I'd read that the first six months after an accident are among the most crucial for rapid repair and threw myself into this. To the ongoing physical, occupational, and speech therapies we added acupuncture, aquatic therapy, massage, chi gong, and an arsenal of supplements and herbs. As the physical breaks healed over, our emotions fractured and conflicts with the children escalated.

Peter's clipped speech and fatigued face conveyed anger he did not always feel. Peter and I undertook some parenting coaching and eventually found the older two children trauma therapists. The children drew pictures of blood and spoke words in anger that I feared, not for what they meant, but for how having said them will weigh on their youth.

Sometimes I wear a ring that came from my mother's family, its band a deep yellow gold set with a diamond and a roughed up sapphire. Letters carved into the inside of its band read EAB to LFW 1930, a gift from my great-great-great grandmother to her son's widow. He died as a medic in the field in WWI and the mourning myth of who he might have become overshadowed future generations. Friends called him Bunty, although that was not his given name. His was one of the first to fill my cup of stories.

As summer gives way to fall, we have moments in which I admire the gold, rubbing against that rich warmth, and others in which all I feel are the sharp ridges left by cracks. A small town jeweler once valued the ring somewhere in the low thousands, but when, in a moment when we had few other means and so many therapies I tried to sell it to a metal trader in the city, he only offered me a few hundred dollars. He'd pull the diamond, dump the sapphire, and melt down the gold, he said, so I'd make the worth of the gold's weight, plus some extra for a diamond cut in the old style. People like a sharper cut these days. And platinum.

If I sold the ring, those initials marking a long ago gift would melt into liquid, joining the gold of other desperate, scorned, or lucky people in a vat. Better to keep it, Peter and I agree and I take to wearing the ring and rubbing its thick art-deco band. On my body sits our last four hundred dollars. I rub and rub the gold with my thumb and it seems to soften with the heat of my hand.

———/———

If I Die Young

Rianne Palazzolo

"Good-bye, Dominic! I love you and I know things will be great," I say as I hug my older brother goodbye. He grabs his bags and turns toward the employee lane of the airport security line. He has just taken a position with Jet Blue as a flight attendant, a job he has dreamed about for years. As he fades into the crowd, I wipe a tear. People look at me as I cry and I realize they probably think we are a couple. It wouldn't be an odd thought as we look nothing alike. I'm petite at 5'1 with olive skin, big brown eyes, and black hair. Dominic stands at 6'2 with paler skin, lighter hair, and each eye a different color—one green and one blue. I always wanted different colored eyes as a child and often viewed his as synonymous with the two worlds he has had to live between—the world of darkness and the world of light.

Thoughts of my brother and his future overwhelm me as he and airport fade in my rearview mirror. As I imagine him sitting miles above me on an airplane, anticipating training in Dallas for months to come, I think about times in his life when he was broken. So broken, repair seemed impossible.

During my freshman year in college, I was always in a time crunch. I was working long hours and taking a full time course load. Dominic is two years older than I, but I have always felt a responsibility to protect him and take care of his needs. That year, however, I rarely had time to spend with him. My phone rang early in the morning on Saturday September 14th, 2010—a date it is easy for me to return to as if it were all happening again.

"Rianne. You need to get to Dominic's. He called me. He's hysterical. I think he has hurt himself," my dad said. I slam my embarrassing flip phone shut and grab my ID. I feel sick to my stomach as I dial Dominic's cell from inside my car.

"Rianne," he sobs. "I am so sorry. I am just . . . so . . . sorry Rianne," he cries uncontrollably.

"I'm on my way to your house. Don't do anything, okay?" I plead as I hang up and try to focus on the road. The sound of my blinker matches my speeding heart rate. After what feels like forever, I am finally on the highway. The speed limit is 70, but I am going at least 80. I have to save Dominic from whatever is happening, and Conway isn't close to North Little Rock. My mind wanders in a million directions as I try to explain what might be going on. "Sorry Rianne," he had said. Sorry for what, I wonder. Did he hit his girlfriend? He is possessive of her. Maybe she fought back and he hit her.

My phone begins to buzz uncontrollably.

"Hello dad," I answer.

"Your brother slit his wrists, Rianne. You need to get there." I can hear the concern deep in his voice. I slam the phone shut without a response. I realize that while on the phone, I had taken the wrong exit. Tears of panic flow as I search for my first opportunity to turn around. My phone buzzes as a text from my cousin flashes across the screen that reads "On my way." My dad must have called him too. I finally turn my car around and get going back the right way toward Dominic.

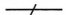

My dad is a gambling addict, and a violent man. As adults, Dominic and I aren't required to deal with him in the same way we did as children, but as our father he still remains a formidable presence. Dominic was such a sweet kid. He has always longed for my dad's approval, love, and affection. I know the tragic events that have unfolded in our lives as they relate to our father contributed to Dominic's emotional damage over the years. He would always suffer a beating when my dad lost a bet. The severity of the beating depended on the amount of money lost. I accepted this reality as a young child because that was just how things went in our home. Dominic also suffered for his own shortcomings. If he struck out at a baseball game, he got beat. If he spilled his orange juice, he got beat. Dominic was an abused child to say the least, and some scenes of his abuse are always fresh in my memory.

One summer day when my mom pulled a double shift, Dominic and I sat arguing over which television show to watch when dad walked through the front door of our home. The brown in his eyes faded into black. He was mumbling under his breath in anger. I glanced at Dominic in a way that suggested we should head to our rooms and we began to creep away. My dad allowed me to pass but jerked Dominic up by his arm. I subconsciously knew this was coming because I had heard my dad cussing the night before about losing $10,000. My stomach turned as I imagined how terrible things were about to get. Dominic began to cry as my dad dragged him into the living room and ordered me to disappear.

The sound was always the worst part. To this day I have never experienced such a helpless feeling as when I heard my brother being beaten. I wanted to help him, to save him. I was too young at age eight to realize the impracticality of saving the world so I just felt guilty. Sometimes even now that I'm in my early twenties, I still feel guilty. Though I was used to the sound by then, this specific instance was different.

I sat on my bed tearing shreds of Kleenex into pieces small enough to fit inside of my ears. I was desperate to drown out the sound of Dominic begging for mercy. After fifteen minutes or so, the sound of his crying stopped. I could still hear the slaps of the belt against his flesh though. I was too afraid to walk out and look. As much as I wanted to save Dominic, I was selfish and didn't want to get in trouble. I crawled on all fours toward the living room to take a peek. Dominic was just lying there limp as my dad continued beating him. The pain in my stomach was unbearable. I blamed myself for not running out there and offering myself up instead.

My dad finally threw the belt down and picked his keys up from the dining room table and left. I guess I thought maybe he was going to get help. Looking back now, I'm not sure why I didn't call the police. I held Dominic in my arms as tears rolled from his closed eyes. After what seemed like a lifetime, he finally opened them.

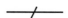

I turn my blinker on as I take the correct exit. Anger flows through all of me. I pull into The Westover Apartments as the American flag moves violently on the pole bolted to a pillar of his apartment building. My cousin David is sitting in his car next to the spot where I park. We walk to the door of Dominic's apartment together.

"Knock on the bathroom door until he responds," David says. David had just tried to go into the bathroom of the apartment but when Dominic didn't respond, he was afraid to walk in alone. In case . . . We take matched, deep breaths and I open the door to the apartment. Never in my life have I been so afraid, so sick to my stomach, so brokenhearted. Part of me thinks he must be dead for sure. And if he is, it is because I took the wrong turn toward Little Rock, adding 20 minutes to the trip. I am sure of that.

" DOMINIC," I scream as loudly as my lungs allow me. " DOMINIC. OPEN. THIS. DOOR. WAKE. UP. NOW," I sob. My world crashes around me. I hit my knees. David stands behind me with his phone set to call 911. In the faintest voice I hear Dominic say "Rianne . . ." I bust into the bathroom to a gut wrenching scene. Blood stains every crevice of the bathroom's tile. I throw up immediately all over the floor. Dominic lies against the bathtub naked and covered in blood. I kneel down and clench his face with my hands. I try to form words as our eyes meet, but none come. I bury my head into his bloody shoulder and cry. On the floor, I see a Yoshi knife our grandmother had bought Dominic, with blood on its blade. Somewhere in my hysteria, I realize that Dominic is still bleeding. I find the words, "Rags. Rags for his wrists. David." David helps me apply pressure to Dominic's freshly slit wrists. We lift him into the shower and begin to cry again as the blood washes away from his body, revealing how pale he is, how much blood he has lost.

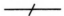

Dominic's iPod plays music through loud speakers on the back of the toilet. "If I Die Young" by The Band Perry is set on repeat. My eyes swell with tears again. I try to refrain from vomiting a second time but can't. At least I make the toilet this time. There is a note next to the iPod dock. It reads: "I, Dominic Angelo Palazzolo, wish to leave everything to my baby sister, Rianne Rae Palazzolo." My mind fixates on Dominic's most recent Facebook post from the morning—a quote from the song now blaring on the radio. *Was he asking for help?* I shiver.

David has Dominic dressed and ready to go. We don't consider cleaning the bathroom. He has stopped bleeding and we decide I can take him to our grandmother's instead of to the ER. We load him in my car and part ways. Dominic sleeps the long ride back to North Little Rock. Long—but not as long as the drive there.

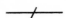

Dominic spent the intervening three years trying to fix himself. He has wanted to be a flight attendant with Jet Blue for forever. He was finally called for an interview April 1, 2014.

"Rianne, guess what!!" he exclaimed. "I'll be joining Jet Blue after all of these years." I am so happy for him, so proud of him. I cry instantly upon receiving the news.

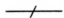

The airport is no longer within sight from my car's rearview mirror. Dominic will claim residence in Dallas for the next three months. He will miss my college graduation. He will be alone.

Dominic is older, but I am stronger. Dominic has always needed and longed for acceptance, and although I, too, long for it from time to time, we need it from different people. When Dominic underwent therapy following his suicide attempt, he always brought up the same idea during sibling sessions. He longs to wake up one day and realize that our entire childhood was a lie. He wants to wake up to a mom who cooks and plays homeroom mother and a dad who pays his taxes and loves his son. For me, this is not appealing. My feelings are that they had their chance to love their beautiful, smart children, and missed out. The loss is theirs.

I feel all of the guilt I've carried for Dominic's childhood settle between my shoulders from time to time. Its presence can overwhelm me. I often wrap my hands around my small wrists, imagining I have scars that match the ones Dominic made visible that day so long ago, scars that now scream survival. Stories between us always contain some sort of selfish act on my part. As I sit down on my couch in silence after dropping him off at the airport, I can't help but pray that this position will work out. I don't pray for this only because it's the natural thing to do. I pray for this because part of me hopes that his happiness will release me. Release me from feeling shackled, from feeling responsible, from feeling suffocated.

On rainy days, and on cold days, and on Dominic's birthday, and sometimes every day of the week, I think back to the summer Dominic was beaten unconscious and how I did nothing to stop my dad. I think back to taking the wrong exit, the day I almost lost Dominic forever, and how I didn't call the police to get to him sooner. I think about the sadness he has endured and the suffering he has survived. Today, though, I think about his future and how bright it is as the sun finally rises to shine on him. I think about never realizing how much you love someone—so much it hurts—until you stand within seconds of losing them, even if only to a new apartment in Dallas.

———/———

Cut

Chelsey Clammer

There is the decision to cut. It is not a decision. There is a need, and there is a want to make that need go away. To simultaneously want to and not want to cut. How the want is an addiction. I want to talk about the cutting because from all of the stares I get, I know you want to know. And this is what I know: the cutting gives you both a sense of control and also the feeling of letting go. And once I started cutting, I did not want to stop. No, I did want to stop, but couldn't.

It started with a sense that there was a space between my veins and my skin I had to get to, had to see what was missing, had to understand what wasn't quite fitting. I needed to see what was in there, what was making my skin feel so unattached from my body, from the tissue that lies underneath. I grabbed a razor and tried to find out. Tried to cut deep in order to carve out that emptiness inside of me. What came up was blood. And when I licked it (*yes, licked it*) the iron tasting liquid momentarily subsided its flow to show translucent flesh mixed with a few globs of yellow—the layer of fat underneath the skin.

---/---

Anatomy of skin.

The skin is the body's largest organ as it covers the entire body. In addition to serving as a protective shield against heat, light, injury, and infection, the skin also regulates body temperature and stores water and fat. There are three primary layers to the skin. The epidermis is what you can see, the hardened outer layer that does not contain any blood vessels. If you cut through the epidermis, you will run into the dermis. This is the chunk of skin through which the blood vessels, the nerves, and the muscles run. Cut even farther down, and you hit the subcutaneous fat layer. Here, it is yellow. Here, the flesh turns pulpy and soft, here there is more blood and more nerves.

My skin did not protect me against injury. As I cut, I went through the epidermis and the dermis, and I could see down into the subcutaneous layer, the pulpy clouds of yellow billowing up. All of me was there, all of that skin layered on top of itself, covered in blood and nerves. I was searching for that empty space I thought I felt, searching for what was missing. I never found what was missing. And each morning I woke with pieces of torn fabric tied to my skin, an outer layer of cloth to keep what was bleeding buried, hidden from the world, known only to me. Finding myself covered in a fresh flesh wound, I still felt lost, I still knew nothing.

I cut in many places. Not just across the geography of my skin—arms, wrists, hands, fingers, hips, stomach, ankles, legs—but in different locations as well. Cutting is about ritual, about a mounting anticipation, about the excitement that you know what's about to come. And then it comes—that incredible calm as you put your tools in place and prepare the setting.

First there was my room. The one on Newgard with the cracked windows Scotch taped together. I hid my instruments in my top dresser drawer. The razor, the navy blue fabric strips, the white gauze and surgical tape. But soon staying in the confines of my room wasn't enough. I craved the cut throughout the day, so I created a traveling kit. A green padded pouch filled with a small razor removed from a surprisingly sharp pencil sharpener, and Band-aids. At work, I would slip into the bathroom stall, clicking the maroon metal door in place behind me. I would lay out my tools on the top of the toilet, roll up my sleeves, and settle into my ritual. Cut. Lick. Dab the blood with toilet paper. Affix Band-aid. Roll down sleeves. A secret all for me.

The pleasure in cutting wasn't ever about the pain. It was about how I could hide the swipes, control what the world saw of me. And how cutting became a ritual, first the cut, then the covering, then the sight of myself hardening—a scab forming, showing me what could be repaired, what could heal.

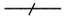

Anatomy of a scab.
When there is a deep wound a clot will form. Blood flow increases and many cells move to the wound. This is how a scab forms, the granulated tissue fills the wound, initiates growth of epithelial cells beneath the scab. The scab will fall off when the skin is regenerated, when it returns to its normal thickness.

After a few weeks, the scab would be ready to be removed, removed as in I could pick it off in mostly one piece. A thin section of dried granulated cells torn away from my body. And when I saw that more skin had regenerated itself underneath, I felt whole for just a second. Enter: anxiety. Anxiety over one whole piece of flesh covering the entirety of my body would settle in, and the addiction to cut into myself, to see what was inside come seeping out—all of it would rise up again. I needed that fix, that secret, that something that was all mine.

I eventually had to get stitches, which was a fascinating adventure. The questions at the hospital: *Are you suicidal?* No. *How old are these scars?* Years. *Did you put all of them there yourself?* Of course. *Do you have a therapist?* Yes.

They never asked if I was drunk.

Because the cutting was done when I was drunk, and it would immediately sober me up. The drink. The ritual. The rush of the cut. Then, at times, the deep gash that led to a hurried drive to the ER. The questions, the assessment, the social worker, then the stitches. Finally, the stitches. The nurses would numb my arm, the skin. Then poke nylon through it and start stitching me back together. I was fascinated by this act, by the ability of the open wound to close in on itself with the assistance of more elements that pierced through the flesh.

———/———

Anatomy of sutures.

There are numerous suture kits in every hospital. Inside the kit are the precise instruments used to suture the skin back together. They are: curved hemostat, sterile scalpel blade, surgical probe, operating and suture lip scissors, pointed forceps, non-suture wound closure strips, tincture of benzoin swabs, antiseptic towelettes, black nylon sutures. Hemostats are scissor-looking clamps that hold onto the skin while the sutures are sewn in. Once the wound is numbed by injecting an anesthetic, the nurse will begin to prepare the sterile instruments to bring the skin back together. While the anesthetic does work, you are still able to feel the pull and tug of the skin surrounding the cut.

The nurses never asked if I could feel it. Perhaps they did not want to know, did not want for me to answer with an ecstatic, *yes.*

I write this story to tell you what it's like to purposefully disfigure your body. To alter your flesh in the way a tattoo does. Only the scars are not celebrated as art. They are tally marks for moments that felt hard.

I do not know why I first started cutting. I had randomly done it as a teenager, a nick here, a small scrape on my wrist, the cuts barely enough to indent my flesh. There were never any scabs, just the flesh as it quickly healed overnight. Think paper cuts. As a teen, I knew that cutting was a way to relieve some inner pain. I don't remember what movies I saw or books I read that lead me onto this notion. But I somehow knew that self-harm was a way to get to it, a way to express that deeper level of pain.

I never tried to burn myself, because, ironically, that sounded painful. And there wouldn't be the blood to see, the layers of epidermis for my eyes to crawl into. I did not want to see my skin pucker up. I wanted to dive into it, to separate it apart in order to find a way in.

As an adult, what started it all were the memories. Memories of a drunken father, an unstable childhood, and a sexual assault in my twenties had all one way or another terrorized my skin, skin that then wanted to crack open in order to let the anxiety over these events seep out.

—————/—————

Anatomy of a cutter.

The behavior of those for whom self-harm is believed to be a morbid form of self-help. For people whose emotions are hyper-reactive or for those raised in an emotionally chaotic environment, cutting or creating physical pain feels like the best way to silence the anxiety, to shut out the memories. After surviving a traumatic situation, a person will often relieve the anxiety that the trauma produced by creating physical harm. Like popping a balloon, the anxiety seems to just go away. For a while.

I do not remember which cut was the first cut, which slowly-forming scar started it all. And I do not know what made me take that first swipe. I know I must have been drunk, as most bad ideas sounded fabulous when I was wasted. So for a few years I made altering my skin a weekly routine. Drink. Cut. Bandage. Scab. Scar. Drink. Cut. Bandage. Scab. Scar. Once a week. Wash. Rinse. Repeat.

And then near the end of my cutting career I cut so badly, again, that I needed to get stitches, again. That would be the fifth time in a year that I had to get stitches. By then, the fascination of it had worn off. I was sick of the questions, the assessments, the social workers. Although watching the suturing of my skin was still interesting. This time, though, I wasn't drunk when I cut, but hungover. I drank the night before. And I cut the night before. When I woke up hungover, bleeding, and in a well of depression, I did what I thought would heal it all, I cut.

And not being drunk, the cut finally hurt.

This has to stop, I screamed at my skin, shouting at the scars, the tallies piled up on my arms.

Hospital, stitches, then off to the psych ward. I was there for ten days, and in those ten days I got sober and stayed sober.

But I did not fully stop the cutting.

In sobriety, the cuts lessened, became smaller. I could fully feel the pain, and it didn't feel relieving, but harsh. The frequency of the cutting faded away long before the scars did. I have fair skin, skin that does not look good dressed in purple clothes, let alone skin that looks good with purple scars snaking up my arms. I had to stop cutting in order to start living, to start enjoying the flesh in which I lived.

How this could end.
I tell you I regret it all, that I look at my eighty-eight scars in horror.

I do not. I see them, and I see me. I have twelve tattoos, and while as an adult I wouldn't get some of them now, I do not regret any of the art. At one point the images were important enough to me to get them permanently imprinted on my body. They are mile markers to me, showing me who I have been. Same with the scars. Those scars were me for three years, were what I identified with. Sometimes, like during job interviews or around my young nieces and nephew, I wish they weren't there, wish that my past pain wasn't published on my flesh. But there is no deleting of this past, no erasing or editing who I have been.

Here is the part on healing.
My skin feels attached now, the hollow somehow removed. Did the cutting do it? No. But the reckoning with the trauma of cutting did. I got sober and got over it. I still live with the scars, but I no longer crave making them. I now yearn to live in this skin, this body, this space I have found and call my own.

Here is the part on reality.
There is a decision to cut. It is not a decision.

Cover Up

Kelli Dunham

My first visit to Haiti was in 1987, a year after the Duvaliers were kicked out and the spring after I turned 18. I went for three months to work as an assistant to a nurse practitioner. I traveled with him to rural clinics, passed out pills, took blood pressures, and changed dressings. I returned to college, but with Haiti in the back of my mind. It was not a place to be forgotten easily.

In 1988, I was in a 17 car pile-up on the way to take the GRE during an ice storm in Oklahoma City. True to midwest values, everyone immediately got out of their cars and started introductions, and then eventually went as a group for hot chocolate at a nearby Dunkin' Donuts while we waited for the highway patrol to come. While the rest of the group was becoming lifelong friends, I was seething over my fake marshmallows. I was missing the last GRE and pretty much ruining my plans to go to graduate school for English and become a teacher and writer. I didn't really have a backup plan, so I decided I could just as well help people while I was figuring out my life. I'd heard about a Haitian school for kids with orthopedic disabilities where volunteers were needed to help run recreational activities for the kids. No special skills were required. I thought, "Well, that's me; I certainly don't have any special skills!" I figured I could devote a month or two while figuring out my next step. I left again for Port au Prince.

I stayed for three years. Haiti is not a place to be let go easily.

At the end of those three years, I left to become a nun. And then, well . . . a lot of things happened. Going to the convent, leaving the convent, coming out, nursing school, and in the mid 90s, although my outer life seemed more situated than it had ever been, my inner life began careening out of control.

I had learned many positive things growing up in a large stoic Germanic farm family: how to get up early and work very hard, how to deny myself current pleasure for future gain, and the difference between a hoe and a backhoe. One thing I didn't learn was how to deal with my feelings. Or really how to recognize that I was having feelings at all. I was the youngest of seven in a family that in many ways was just barely hanging on. In this context, toughness was the most prized attribute of all. Everything, in fact, could be leveraged as a toughness lesson. My siblings and I used to joke that if we came into the house screaming, "The disc [a very sharp farm implement] cut off my thumb and it's out in the yard," my mom would reply, "You march out there and you pick up that thumb. You know we don't leave things lying around like that." This was hyperbole in a technical sense, but emotionally it was not far off at all. With this family canvas as the backdrop to my life, it may not be surprising that the idea of self-soothing seemed like—as my dad would have said— "hippie shit."

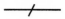

So I began cutting myself.

It's almost impossible to understand now who I was then. How the hell did cutting myself help? But the truth is, it did for a while. Until my upper left arm was a maze of scars and I was having trouble keeping it a secret. Cutting is a habit that scares folks. I knew I had to find some other coping mechanisms.

So, I did.

The scars didn't really bug me that much, not the scars themselves. I couldn't and didn't want to always keep them covered up. Sometimes it'd get hot goddamnit! Also, I happen to really like my shoulders and it's hard to show off one's shoulders except in a sleeveless shirt.

But the scars distracted people. Some people. There were folks who wanted to ask me lots of questions, or even schedule an intervention. For example, despite the fact that the youngest of the scars is maybe fifteen years old, I actually had a therapist follow me around at an outdoor community event one year, telling me, "You know you don't have to live like this. I can help you."

I also had a woman tell me (at a dyke march no less) that I should put my shirt on because seeing my scars was, "Like experiencing an act of violence that makes me feel unsafe."

As to those who would ask questions, I would deflect most queries with a cheery, "It's a long story," and a quick change of the subject. If someone was being mean, judgmental, or intrusive I just smiled as icily as I could, saying slowly, "Everyone. does. what. they. need. to. survive." Many folks who didn't ultimately ask would do a very obvious double take. Sometimes there was judgment in their stares, often there was not. But people noticed, and my scars allowed people to assume that I was in an emotional place that I truly wasn't.

For several years, I considered a cover up tattoo, and even visited several tattoo artists to discuss possibilities. When one refused, saying that they wouldn't ink my scar tissue, I would go on to the next, but I was deflated after several attempts at what was beginning to seem impossible. In 2005, I started dating someone who loved my scars. Once I mentioned to her that a tattoo person had refused to even consider trying a cover-up and her response was, "There's plenty of skin there. Just keep asking until you find someone who's not scared."

This same lover decided I needed some specific tattoo ideas. We both had a bit of a crush on the Virgin Mary especially as she appeared in Lourdes, although we agreed a hippie Mary would look much cooler than an overly angelic one. And then there're roses and, of course because we loved juxtaposition, thorns. I wanted Mary to be at least chunky . . . "She needs to look like she shops at Lane Bryant. At their upper end," was how I explained it later to the tattoo chick.

I finally found someone through a friend who came highly recommended. I made an appointment, told her what I wanted, rolled up my sleeve, and her response was, "Oh, I can do that. Those scars don't scare me." She designed the tattoo within two days, and on the third day she inked me in one sitting. She was totally cool and very skillful. The scars took the ink and that was that. Pretty non-dramatic. And yet for me, huge. And a huge gift.

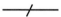

After the earthquake in Haiti in January 2010, I knew I needed to return and do what I could. Haiti is not a place one forgets easily.

I worked at a small field hospital where many of the patients were kids. Because of the way buildings fell, especially in the most populated areas of Port au Prince, and the time of day, as well as their relatively smaller size, kids seemed like they survived more often than adults. We had a number of *Se li min ki te solve* kids. "He was the only one that was saved."

Six year old Emmanuel was one of them. The first day I worked at the hospital, I was pushing IV Ancef—a very potent antibiotic usually given in a less aggressive manner—and trying not to think about how dangerous the practice was when Emmanuel approached me. He had a hefty bandage around his head, a cast on his right leg and another on his left arm, and healing scratches all over.

"I have a problem" he said, literally climbing up the side of me. "My mom and dad are dead."

Because he was clinging very tightly to me, I had little choice but to hold him back as I returned with him hanging on my hip to our temporary "nurses station" (really the kitchen from a converted children's home).

When I stopped walking, Emmanuel looked up at me. "And the rest of my family, too."

I glanced over at the pediatrician who had arrived a few days before me. I mouthed "All his family is dead?" to her. She shook her head. "No. He still has his grandma. So there's someone to send him home to when he's better."

I continued to hold Emmanuel while I prepared the rest of the evening's meds. After that, whenever he asked and I had an extra arm and/or a free lap, he was in it or on it. He became fascinated with my coverup tattoo and constantly asked me to make one for him. I told him that people just can't go around giving tattoos to 7-year-olds, *and* I didn't know how to do tattoos, *and* I didn't have the equipment, *and* his scratches and lacerations were still healing. Still, every day, he asked.

On my last day at our makeshift clinic, my thoughts were torn between Haiti and home. I was using my sharpie to write the change date on an IV bag when I had an idea. I called Emmanuel over and asked him to roll up his sleeve. Using the thick blue marker, around the healing areas of his left upper arm, I drew a very rough form of the Virgin Mary.

Emmanuel regarded his arm, and could not stop smiling.

"*Nou blese mim jam,*" he said. "We have the same wounds"

How do you tell a kid that, no, my post adolescent difficulties in handling my temperamental mismatch with my dysfunctional family of origin does not compare with his loss of his entire family, being gravely injured, and having to heal in a country impoverished by centuries of racism and colonialism?

You can't. Not when he's just said, "We have the same wounds"

So I picked him up and said, "*Enben, verman, vre, nou cou-vre-yo mim jam.*" "Well, we definitely cover them up the same way."

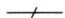

Beast Within

Michelle Jarvis

I have never had a positive body image. The adolescent awkwardness of having a body that developed on its own schedule, a schedule unlike and ahead of my friends', never quite left me. Then, middle age and gravity added their own special indignities. Before my cancer diagnosis at forty-four, it had been more than a decade since I had felt anything other than fat and old and ugly. For the most part, I was able to keep my body image separate from my sense of self-worth, but my negative body image was always there, lurking like a caged beast, waiting to be unleashed.

That isolated beast gained strength from the cancer when I added an incision that has been opened over the same surgical line three times and extends from just above my pubic bone to below my sternum, several drain scars, an ileostomy scar, and (worst of all) a permanent colostomy. The ileostomy, a diversion of the intestinal tract where the small intestine is pulled through the abdominal wall and culminates with a plastic bag to capture the intestinal contents, was always planned to be temporary to allow the colon to heal after surgery. However, when the colon was resected and the two remaining ends connected, the connection failed, necessitating emergency surgery that resulted in a permanent colostomy. Now, the colon—instead of the small intestine—is pulled through the abdominal wall and ends with a plastic bag to capture the fecal output of the colon. My midsection is a mess, and my life will never be the same.

The indignity of emptying my colostomy bag's contents several times a day is bad enough, but it comes with other less-than-lovely bonuses. When my bag is full of output or bloated with gas, it bulges, causing unsightly and embarrassing protrusions under clothing, especially under sheer clothing such as underwear and lingerie. Swimwear is a challenge, and even everyday clothes cause me to check my appearance constantly, fearing others will notice what I know is present.

———/———

I get the "gross" factor. I really do. If for nothing other than the unpleasantness of it all, I understand that my new body is one that most people don't care to see. I also understand that my new body can be hard to face for my loved ones, not because they are repulsed, but because it is difficult to confront the evidence of the pain and fear I have faced. I don't force my new body upon anyone, except my spouse.

For a while, I felt as if my body were public domain because so many medical professionals had poked and prodded the most private nooks and crannies of it. Because I was so ill, my husband saw and attended to more of my bodily needs than I care to name. When it came to my body as a private, sensual and sexual entity, life would never be the same. Finding intimacy again is difficult when your body no longer seems to be your own.

Cancer, any cancer, is an assault on femininity. Most people can understand how breast cancer and gynecological cancer can destroy a woman's sense of femininity. Culturally, missing breasts are an overt sign of diminished womanhood, and the absence of female reproductive organs causes a host of unwomanly features to appear. Perhaps because of the attention drawn to these cancers, people have grown to understand how they can impact femininity and to some degree understand how devastating they can be for a woman's self-image. But this is not true of colon cancer. The effects of colon cancer are more hidden, harder for a culture to process and embrace.

Colon cancer is generally perceived as a disease that impacts the digestive system, not one that impacts life as a woman. In my case, that perception couldn't be more wrong. A hysterectomy was needed to resect the colon, and the long hair I had treasured for all my life thinned and shortened during treatment. My nails cracked and fell off, and my skin erupted in a rash before drying to scales. Scar tissue in the abdomen constricted the vagina, causing pain during sex in addition to the other unpleasantries of radiation induced menopause. None of this helped me to find my sexuality again or to quell the nagging beast of poor body image.

I tried to buy my way out of inadequate femininity. I bought clothes with fold-over waists and tight, stretchy hips that would support and conceal my colostomy bag. I bought a black, spaghetti-strap nightie and a matching ruched black intimacy band with tiny red bows to cover the colostomy during intimate moments, in case they ever happened again. I bought cute lacy panties, full enough to cover the worst of the scarring but sheer enough to be seductive. They made me feel feminine, sexy even.

Sexy—until I asked my husband to take a peek. He couldn't look. I was crushed. The only person who mattered to me couldn't bear the sight of my new body. How would we heal this scar? Friends told me not to worry, that there were other ways to be intimate, but I wasn't convinced. My husband is, after all, still a man. No situation could be any more intimate than those we had faced during my illness, but sex had become foreign.

The solution was time, lots of time. And my time schedule wasn't his time schedule. I knew my body, and I knew when the internal and external scars were ready to find the new normal, but he didn't, and he had scars of his own. He needed time to overcome the fear that he would hurt me. He needed time to stop being a caregiver and start being a husband again.

Sex still isn't easy, and it might never be again. The work might not be worth it. I don't know, but I'm willing to keep working, for now.

Most days, I can live with all of this, the bag and even the scars, in part because I have to, and in part because I believe the scars mean something more than just disfigurement. They are battle scars that came from winning a hard-earned victory. They are symbols of life and hope that are more important than the scars themselves. They are reminders that the beast can be tamed.

———/———

WRITTEN IN STITCHES

Samantha Plakun

Five pearly inches across
the curve of my abdomen,
Or twelve centimeters
and 7/10 of another.

Writing on my body
that keeps my insides sewn up
and from falling out
onto cool linoleum floors.

Telling our story
like cursive on a carcass.
Something I will always have
to stand behind.

The first time I saw you,
we were alone.
On a bare day
I could feel you,

underneath my hospital gown.
We took it slow,
afraid of the warm
sensation between skin and tape.

And in that naked light
you were disgusting.
There was no comfort to be found
in gauze or surgical string.

At home on my already imperfect relic, a hypertonic trophy.
A way out of work, an excuse to play hooky,
both buttress and gargoyle;
support and grotesque protection.

We grew into each other
like conjoined twins.
My closeness with another becomes
our closeness with another.

"How'd you get that?"
And we might as well be alone.

———/———

PERMANENT MARKER

Aimee Ross

I stand naked on a wooden box in the meat-locker cold of the plastic surgery prep room, where two nurses watch the plastic surgeon mark up my body with a black sharpie.

He is sitting on a stool on wheels, eye-level with my abdomen, and he leans forward, drawing slowly. He pauses, rolls backward with his heels, and takes in the surgical map of my front in its entirety.

I'm freezing, and I self-consciously wonder if he notices my erect nipples. If he does, he doesn't show it. Instead, he moves forward again and resumes the process of grabbing skin, charting lines, and scrutinizing the results. He takes his time, but I can't fault him. I want him to go slow. I want him to make sure the markings are perfectly placed.

In a few moments, he will be cutting those lines and "revising" the scar that runs the length of my torso. The scar that was made to save my life two years before.

Actually, I have more than ten scars all over my body from that night. Places where bones punctured skin, where chest tubes inflated lungs. Where a seatbelt held me fast. Where crushed, sharp metal scored skin. Where an eight-inch plate braces a snapped humerus and a three-inch pin secures a fractured pelvis. Where wires and screws hold a dislocated foot in place. Where IVs found the perfect veins to tap.

Some of the scars are short, some are long, some are hard to see. Almost all of them are vertical.

At right angles to a horizontal plane. Perpendicular.

The same angle at which we collided when he ran that stop sign and into my car, t-boning it and me.

My vertical scars, the places I was put back together, stitched back up.

And none of them compares to the disfiguring scar running straight up my abdomen. The scar I worry people can see through my clothing. The scar that hurts to the touch.

—— / ——

I hate this fucking scar.

—— / ——

"Should I try to save your belly button?" he pulls the permanent marker away from my flesh and looks up long enough to ask.

I am surprised by the option. I doubt anyone would consider it a navel as it is, smashed up and pushed away from its point of origin.

"No, it's okay," I answer, and he continues on with his design.

Two years before, trauma doctors had not asked me what to save. They had not planned the carved path their knife would take, nor did they plot the route around my belly button. They were trying to save my life. They just cut.

"We had to have them do *that*— " my brother said as he pointed to my abdomen "—to be able to have you here now."

That.

I could almost picture *it*. Me, unconscious and naked, blue paper medical drapes covering legs and arms, breasts and belly exposed. Me, flat on a stainless steel table in a cold operating room, where white lights radiate and whispery instructions intensify. A quick surgical cut, the flash of blade piercing flesh, just above the sternum down down down around the umbilicus down through to the pubis.

Done. That quick. A way to get inside.

Internal bleeding and lacerated organs and a ruptured spleen. My body left open for the bleeding to stop and the swelling to lessen, then closure of muscle tissue only, a wound vac in place. The vacuum pump removed excess fluid as it increased blood flow to heal the wound from the inside out until the outside could be surgically closed.

But I didn't want *that* surgery. It was my fault.

Dr. Yowler, that too-jovial trauma doctor, gave me a choice—leave the wound vac in or be closed up—six of one, or half dozen of another, he said. But I said no. I didn't want another surgery, so the vacuum stayed in. For almost three months.

Maybe I should have gone back under the knife now that I think about it. That scar couldn't have been worse than this one.

This monstrous scar, gaping, still tender two years later. I think about the accident every time I get dressed. I cry every time I see myself naked.

Doctors assured me the wound would grow together on its own, but no one could tell me what the scar might look like. I imagined a normal, smooth surgical scar. Surely, I believed, since they had cut me straight, my belly would mend together that way, too.

But it didn't.

When the skin of my abdomen was finally closed three months later, a messy, uneven, and ugly scar ran its length: a ten-inch long ribbon undulated from just above my ribcage to just above my pubic bone. Thick, new pink skin stretched wide like a yawn, bridging the fingertip-deep crevice to smooth the fault line of my abdomen's landscape. The ruched tissue puckered in places and pulled in others, dividing my tummy, splitting subcutaneous fat, then narrowed to semi-thick closures at both ends.

What a poetic description.

Let's be real.

The scar makes me look as if I have another ass, but this one is in front. I still have my belly button, but it's scrunched up, almost closed, and pushed to the side, forgotten. The entire area still hurts to the touch because the tissue of my abdomen was so deeply bruised. My clothes even fit differently. I shop for maternity tops—twelve years after my last child was born.

—— / ——

I hate this fucking scar.

—— / ——

The plastic surgeon draws huge circles on my flanks, what he calls the areas of skin just under the ribs and above the waist, where he will also perform liposuction. Then he traces dotted vertical lines around the scar and around my smashed up navel, along with another line, horizontal this time, from hipbone to hipbone. I know this is for the tummy tuck—another scar to add to the canvas.

He finishes with his magic marker, and I step down from the box and look in the mirror, avoiding his and the nurses' eyes. I have never been completely naked in front of this many people before—at least not awake—and I am embarrassed by my nudity. All of my flaws have been highlighted by a map of black ink stretching across the flesh of my tummy. Somehow, I understand this strange picture. The skin around my scar will be cut away, the rest pulled together, smoothed tight, and stitched closed. The disfigurement will be corrected, the excess fat and extra skin discarded.

In my head, I say a quick prayer: **Please God, let opening my body again bring closure.**

"Okay," he says, tucking the pen into his pocket, slapping the palms of his hands on his thighs. "It's time! I'll see you when you wake up."

In the next few hours, this plastic surgeon will do what others said they couldn't do. He will revise the lumpy, raw scar gaping across my belly into a smooth, flesh-colored, skinny seam, one that will be unexpectedly beautiful. He will join it with the new scar, the one from hip to hip, and together they will form what looks like an anchor.

An anchor: the steadfast support I will need to allow the old scar to transform to mere memory. To become the history of *my* story.

He smiles.

"You'll be great, Aimee," he reassures me, and I know in that moment that he is the one who will be great, not me.

His permanent mark on my abdomen will be the seal of a clean slate, the promise for peace of mind and an improved body. For this, I will be forever grateful.

It's time.

———/———

COLLIDE

Douglas Kidd

The accident was on May 17, 2005. As I experienced states of either coma or amnesia for more than two months, I have no memories of that day. The crash occurred when an SUV travelling roughly fifty miles per hour smashed into my Acura Integra (Figure 1). Photographs of the vehicles set on a collision course that day prove what I cannot recall.

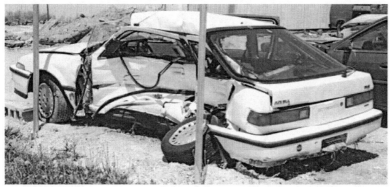

Figure 1

Of course, I am extremely fortunate to have survived the ordeal, and the event altered me in profound ways. In addition to multiple internal injuries, hip fractures, and a crush injury to my lower right leg which led to compartment syndrome (increased pressure in a muscle compartment that can lead to muscle and nerve damage as well as blood flow problems), the concussive forces of the collision caused the most significant injury when my brain hemorrhaged severely.

While physical aspects of the scars healed long ago, they are direct evidence of past events and serve daily to evoke memories, reflection, and emotion.

First, I will point you to my largest and longest scar. The scar tapers to nearly half an inch deep, is one inch at its widest, and travels nearly 12 inches along the shin of my right leg (Figure 2). Evidently, as the SUV collided with the driver's side of my car, the forces of the collision threw my leg violently to the right, pinning it against the transmission covering, causing my leg to burst open. Later, as I lay in my hospital bed with eyes closed or unfocused, my brain attempted to process my surroundings. The constant noise and smell from the medical device that surrounded my leg greatly assisted the beginning of my reconnection to the world. Memories of that machine working on my leg during my reawakening have faded now, but I dimly recall being irritated by the device as it made an incessant thrumming, reminiscent of summer nights when cicadas fill the air with

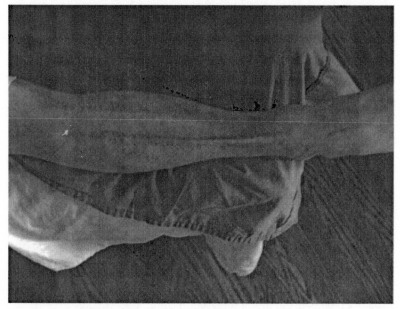

Figure 2

their noise. The smell made by the device as it removed fluids from my healing leg was like rotting garbage. These medical treatments to save my leg were among the first sources of stimulation welcoming me back to life.

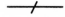

As my recovery progressed, I received twice-daily medical treatments to replace the bandages on my lower right leg that became saturated with blood and to dress the open wound. Usually, one treatment came in the morning and another in the evening. Of course, I was anchored by heavy doses of morphine, which I could self-administer by depressing a hand-held device. I recall while the effect of the drug lasted, the injury was not overly painful. As the days passed, out of concern for the narcotic and highly addictive side effects of the morphine, doctors gradually weaned me from the drug. I do recall that the ache of pain from my leg increased as the medication decreased, but given the excitement of my developing ability to re-engage the world around me, this concern faded to the background. I was grateful for the treatment sessions as they afforded me opportunities to socialize with hospital staff. During one session, a nurse's assistant could not get over the size of the scar and openly wondered how I managed to keep my leg. It is interesting to note that I do not experience stigma, which to me is closely tied to shame, associated with this scar on my leg. In fact, during warmer months, I am unafraid to reveal this scar to others and I usually wear shorts. Regardless of the outside temperature, when travelling by air, I've found shorts make it more comfortable in cramped seating spaces and I always boldly display this scar.

A few years ago, I had interesting experiences in connection with this scar on flights to and from London. In Detroit following the return flight, I deplaned and headed to customs. As I approached the queue for re-admission processing to the United States, an official noticed my scar. He gestured towards my leg and said the scar looked "incredibly painful" and asked if I required a wheeled chair. I said no thank you and proceeded towards the back of the line. However, he intervened and directed me to a much shorter line for either elderly passengers or those using wheeled chairs. What is more, the official—much to the consternation of a woman in her sixties—placed me squarely in front of her in the line and promptly left. This led to a few awkward and uncomfortable moments talking with the woman as I explained I did not request the special service the official initiated, and apologized for cutting in front of her. However, my placement in the front of the line meant that I was soon out of the airport and on my way.

A similar experience occurred on the flight over to London where an immigration official noticed my scar and directed me to an expedited queue. While I was not directed to the head of this line, I did have a much shorter wait than ordinary travelers. It is interesting to note, upon seeing my scar on both occasions, immigration officials immediately responded as if something were wrong. Of the several disfigurements I possess, while the scar on my lower right leg is certainly dramatic and even a little frightening to see, it neither causes me difficulty, nor does it limit my life. However, the scar signals to others something is unusual and potentially wrong. In the two examples described above, people perceived the difference my scar presents and responded positively out of concern for me, then sought to improve my condition.

In contrast to confidently displaying my leg disfigurement, I am perhaps overly sensitive to revealing the scar on my neck, which was once an opening to accommodate a tracheostomy tube (Figure 3). While in ICU, I was unable to breathe on my own. At first, I was intubated with a tube extending through my mouth and into my lungs. However, among other aspects that were signals of my early recovery—responding to various sensory stimuli and opening my eyes—to better accommodate me as I became more active, and yet permit the ventilator to function, a tracheostomy tube fitting was installed in my throat. Also, restraints were in place as I was disoriented following the coma with no awareness of my circumstances.

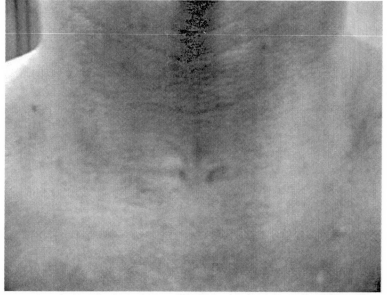

Figure 3

Family reminds me that towards the end of my stay in ICU, I actively resisted my restraints and physically challenged the medical personnel who took care of me. On one such occasion (I was unaware of my actions at the time and do not recall the incident now), I managed to rip the tracheostomy tube from my throat and actually attempted to get out of bed. I try to imagine my limited ability to process the world at the time, and I must have thought, *Where am I? What is this tube in my throat? It is not me and I want no part of it!* As I reflect on that moment now, perhaps dimly remembering my time spent in restraints, emotions flood over me. An image forms of me lying in a hospital bed seriously injured with tubes and machines attached to me as I fight for my life; yet for my own safety, I am restrained. These images provoke memories that sometimes produce an overwhelming sense of helplessness, desperation, isolation, and loss, where all I can process is tears. It is odd that such a small thing as the scar on my neck sometimes triggers significant emotional collapses.

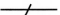

I name the scar for the tracheostomy tube as "star shaped" because it vaguely resembles a crude drawing a child might make to represent a star. It is difficult to express the precise reasons for my sensitivity to displays of this scar. As I reflect, it seems as if my concerns primarily center on perceptions of how I and others interpret the scar. On the one hand, the scar on my leg is roughly one hundred times larger than the scar on my throat. So, clearly size is not the stigmatizing issue. The scar on my leg does signify I have come through extraordinary circumstances that somehow distinguish me from others, and this feeds my positive self-image. Whereas the scar in my throat, because of its location, does signify a near-facial disfigurement, and I am uncomfortable revealing it to others. Early in my recovery, I used to display the tracheotomy scar; but as I became more aware of my surroundings, and sensitive to the feedback demonstrated by stares, I find myself uncomfortable, and do all I can to eliminate this feeling. I hide this scar. I manage to conceal it by using a shirt's top button, or in colder months I wear a turtleneck. Some may consider this odd behavior, but unless you've experienced the uncomfortable stares from people, it is difficult to anticipate how you might respond.

Another stigmatizing scar is more than a quarter inch wide and nearly eleven inches long on the center of my abdomen. I can only speculate as to reasons for the scar; I had several major internal injuries, such as a liver laceration and ruptured spleen, which developed in response to the forces of the collision as I was thrown violently against my shoulder restraint. Also, below my navel, the scar deepens, widens, and becomes more pronounced. Stigma that I associate with this abdominal scar is the reason that unless it is a rare day spent swimming or at a beach, I always conceal it from view. Conspicuously, even in an essay in which scars are the subject, I am reluctant to expose this scar to others and even to myself. I have thoughts of one day having surgery on my abdominal and throat scars to improve their appearance. In contrast, I have never entertained ideas of having plastic surgery on my leg.

The scars I have sometimes evoke direct responses from others. Based on these interactions, it is my considered opinion that scars are like canvases on which people project their ideas—sometimes fears—of human difference. It is human nature to be curious about encounters with the unknown and the unexpected. It seems as sentient organisms, we are hard-wired to perceive difference, so that we might potentially respond to threats to our continued existence. Scars are clear indicators of human difference. What is more, scars often lower the barrier that exists to define the limits of ordinary human interactions. For example, as I waited outside the Metropolitan Museum of Art in New York, a woman in her early twenties made me feel very uncomfortable as she stared at the scar on my leg for nearly ten minutes. What is more, after a time, she broke the usual silence that exists among strangers in the city, when she asked if I were in pain. I will give her the benefit of the doubt and assume she was expressing genuine concern for me, but I believe she was also responding to the difference my scar signifies, which perhaps she felt empowered her to probe. I responded to her politely, "No, I am not in pain, just waiting for a friend."

It is difficult to guess the motivations of others as they respond to scars I possess. Their concerns may be heartfelt. However, as a former non-disabled person, I have the benefit of remembering my own thoughts and attitudes toward those with physical differences before my accident. I recall having to make a conscious effort not to ask personal questions of those with physical disfigurements. To be honest, I also remember times when some individuals with significant scar damage repelled me. Concern over their scars made it difficult to recognize their humanity and their appearance did not encourage me to engage them in conversation. It seemed as if all positive attributes they possessed were secondary to my irrational concerns over the potential threats they might pose. I can state that in my own experience of scars, I have a newfound awareness of people and recognize scars do not define the individual and say nothing about their humanity.

I have never seen the scars on my brain, nor has anyone, except, I suppose, the neurosurgeons or emergency room personnel in scans created to evaluate the severity of my brain injury; but the concussive forces of the collision caused the appearance of small tears to brain tissues and my brain subsequently hemorrhaged. Some of these scars were to the emotion centers of my brain and this brain damage is expressed by wide swings of emotion. In significant ways, these scars will never heal and can produce emotional inward journeys. Notable and at times sudden expression of emotion is the salient issue I have confronted during my recovery. And, it is ironic these profound emotional outbursts arise from the physically smallest injuries I acquired in the accident. I feel it necessary to relate that these emotional "outbursts" almost always come in the form of emotional collapse. On rare occasions, I have expressed anger, but this anger comes in the form of yelling and never results in physical altercations with others.

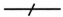

Other scars that I've never seen are to the acetabulums and surrounding tissues of both hips. The ball end of the femur combines with the socket area of the pelvic bone, and together they comprise the acetabulum. Evidently, as my body absorbed the tremendous energies of the SUV, my hips shattered. Scans taken today would reveal many fractures to the dense bones of both femurs and pelvis, the cartilage covering these bones, and tears to the surrounding muscles of my hips. Early in my recovery, I was slated to have hip replacement surgery, but I developed the deadly methicillin-resistant staphylococcus aureus staph infection, more commonly known as MRSA, so the inevitable hip replacement surgery will wait. My mind retains no memory of this time, but visitors had to clad themselves in rubber garments and use respirators to shield me from contracting additional infection. I learned later, it is principally because I developed MRSA and survived that hospital staff called me "the miracle man."

The last consultation I had with an orthopedic surgeon was more than seven years ago. He showed me images of both hips that revealed many fractures to the bones and cartilage that healed to form scars. I asked the doctor how I would know when the surgery is required. He responded in one ominous and scary word: "Pain." These scars on and around my hips remain with me unseen, but from time to time, principally dependent upon the weather, they make me aware of their presence in the form of a dull ache. The scars to my hips indicate that on some future day, I will go under the knife again and create new scars.

Most of this essay is based on reflecting about occurrences from the relatively distant past. However, when I began this writing project, I did not anticipate how re-reading my essay with suggestions from the editor could lead me to reflect on my scars and bring my experiences of accident, injury, and recovery to the present. By engaging in this reflexive process, a flood of uncontrollable emotion ensued. While certainly irrational, as I read the editor's feedback, the amount of time that transpired since the accident seemed to disappear, and it is if I were back in my hospital bed, restrained, confused, disoriented, and in pain. This irrational compression of time and intensity of reliving the experience is an expression of the brain injury I acquired. Remembering my experiences this way became too much for my rational mind to contain, and tears flowed. Some of the tears came from recognition of how far I have come and how drastically altered my life is since the accident. Some of the tears came with an appreciation for simply being alive and the opportunity to have problems to resolve. Unless one has experienced dramatic shifts that come with establishment of a new identity following a significant brain injury, or other life-changing event, it is difficult to appreciate the value of tears; but my experiences have taught me to cherish life and the opportunity to relive my experiences through the memories that are not lost.

From our earliest days, most of us gradually acquire skills to navigate our world, yet when this stream of days that build our autonomy is rudely interrupted, the chasm of confusion and despair that opens beneath our feet is overwhelming. What may be surprising is I have come to treasure experience from my emotional side. As is evidenced by the crying episode that emerged during the writing of this essay, the brain damage I acquired in the accident is a scar that is likely to be a source of potential emotional upset that may surface occasionally, and for the rest of my life. But, truly, I am okay with this. As evidence, every May 17 I engage in a small celebration. It may seem unusual and strange to celebrate the anniversary of the most calamitous day of my life, but it is the journey back from oblivion that I treasure, and having the opportunity to appreciate life and my relationships makes me happy. It is not too much to state: since the journey of my life became radically altered by the car accident, I am a new and better person. And, it is the emergence of this person and possibilities for a new life that I celebrate with tears of joy.

I've been informed the car accident occurred because I was distracted by engaging in a cellphone conversation. I have no memory of this occurrence, but evidently, after halting briefly at a stop sign, I proceeded into an intersection without looking closely for cross traffic, when the SUV struck me. More than two years later, shortly after I regained the ability to drive, I found myself answering my cell phone while on my way to work at the university. Seconds after the phone rang and I answered, I ended the conversation. Seconds after that, I found a safe place to stop my car. As soon as I stopped, my entire body shuddered. I said to myself, "Douglas, you have been down that road before. You know how it will end. What are you doing?" Since that day, nearly seven years ago now, I have never used a cell phone while driving. My opposition to using cell phones while driving led me to form a company whose mission is to end this entirely avoidable possibility from occurring to others.

And so, many could say that a greater good has come from my tragedy of May 17, that healing scars have given me a new life, or at least a different understanding of and greater appreciation for the life I am lucky to still have. But they have also left me more open, more exposed to raw emotional experiences, the very sight of my scars forcing me to create and recreate who I am.

Cellular:
An Interview with Lorrie Fredette

Thursday, October 9, 2014

Via Email by Erin Wood

Most of your work relates to aspects of the body unseen by the naked eye. Why do you seek to magnify these hidden parts, in some installations even creating them to fill up the room?

I'm interested in the juxtaposition of the micro (cellular) to the macro (our bodies) and in inverting the relationship so that we perceive our physical bodies as micro in relation to the work.

Unlike your other work (much of which depends on magnification), scars are typically quite visible. So why scars? How, why, and when did you become interested in exploring scars through your work?

Skin is like a canvas of our identity and personality. It naturally shows our age, health, ancestry, and cultural identity. We further modify it through piercings, tattoos, and scarification. When I was introduced to scarification, I became curious about why people would subject themselves to such an experience.

In many indigenous cultures, scarification is part of a ritual of transition from childhood or adolescence into adulthood. Some cultures see this body marking as a sign of beauty. Learning about these tribal rituals and aesthetics made me reflect on the possible histories behind physical scars in our own culture, which doesn't participate in ceremonial scarring. Yet even though we don't use scarring rituals to mark life passages, our scars are visible markers of events that change us permanently, dividing our lives into "before" and "after." We will never again be the unscarred person, the person to whom the event did not happen.

With a few exceptions, we acquire our scars unwillingly, often in horrific circumstances. Our society primarily associates scarring with trauma, certainly not with beauty. Scars, and the painful memories they evoke, are almost always visible to the individual who bears them. But by nature or training, we avert our eyes when someone else's scar is visible; we don't wish to participate in resuscitating the experience that caused the scar.

93

I've been violating that taboo, collecting images of scars by asking family, friends, and acquaintances if they would mind if I photographed their wound(s).

You call your scar works "scar portraits." How did you decide on this term?

Each scar is unique. Each person's scar is distinctive to that individual— not just in the shape, color, and texture of the mark but in the narrative that produced it. Thus, it is a portrait of their body and their history.

I actually see all of my work as a type of portraiture. Each piece refers to the physical body in some way, whether it be a scar, a cell, or a virus.

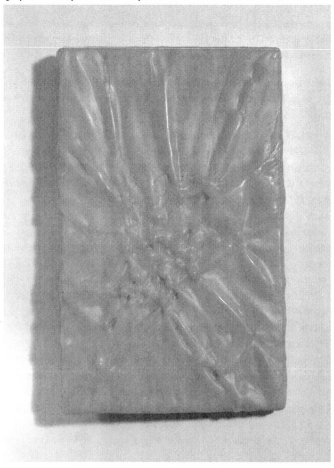

They are often representations of us as individuals and at times, of family, community, or cultural stories. These are all aspects of traditional portraiture.

How did you choose beeswax and tree resin for your series of "scar portraits"? Do you see those mediums having more to do with scars in the process of their construction or the final product? Or neither of those? Something else?

My portfolio contains two bodies of scar works. Beeswax and resin are the primary materials in *Overgrowing the Boundaries*. The most significant historical association of wax is that paraffin has traditionally been used to preserve biological samples. The connotation of "preserving" an abstraction of a scar walks a fine line between intrigue and perversity.

I make the sutured drawings known as *battle lines* from silicone and nylon line. As a practical matter, the materials must meet the physical needs of making the work, and have visual impact. Metaphorically, we think of silicone as a substance we implant in the body, a foreign agent, which has an abstract relationship to the "foreign" body of keloid scar tissue. The nylon line that refers to sutures crosses several visual and cultural layers: the reference to stitching on a representation of the body; and the fact that even today, sewing is often considered women's work.

You called your suture pieces "drawings." I guess a lay person might label them as sculpture. Why "drawings"?

Though each element—the scar, the nylon line, and the paper—are objects, combined they are marks on paper and thus drawings.

What has taken you down the path of working with sutures?

Because of my interest in the landscape of the body, the topography of the skin, I began to consider how it heals. Of course, one way to accelerate healing, often a necessary prerequisite to healing, is the act of suturing a wound. I began to consider the word "suture." Sew. A uniting of parts. While the act of suturing aids the process of healing, that only happens on the physical level. You can't suture the experience, the memory, the narrative. Medical sutures are either snipped off or dissolve once the wound has healed. By leaving the sutures in place in these drawings, I keep alive the question of what happened. The sutures suggest the story of the wound waiting to be told.

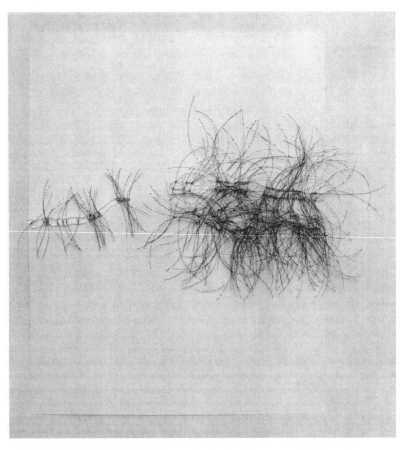

I'd imagine few people other than physicians or veterinarians (and perhaps the patients removing them from their own bodies when necessary) have the opportunity to work with sutures. How does it feel physically to work with sutures? And how do you work physically with them? Any special tools or techniques?

Since some of my training is in textile processes, I'm able to replicate the knots in suturing. Between a used book from 1956 (*Basic Surgical Skills: A Manual with Appropriate Exercises*) and medical YouTube videos, I taught myself the process. In this day and age, I'm guessing that anyone who wants to know how to suture can learn just as I did. The YouTube videos alone would do the trick. My tools were simple: nylon line, a sewing needle, a pair of pliers, and scissors. I started by practicing on oranges.

Since I wasn't suturing any flesh, I didn't need a forceps, a curved needle, a needle holder, or gloves.

To my eye, your suture pieces have an element of creepiness, almost like one of those poisonous fuzzy black caterpillars. They seem to be in motion, or paused momentarily but gaining momentum to move. Is this intentional, or just part of working with this medium (maybe it happens naturally with something that is slick and black)?

Thank you for acknowledging the momentum in these drawings. The pieces where most of the sutures have gone awry tend to demonstrate the most movement. That is most definitely intentional. The combination and interaction of the individual lines enhances the chaos and commotion.

Do you have scars of your own? Has/how has your work changed your views about living with scars?

Yes, I had a "not paying attention" accident and came very close to having a permanent scar. At the time, I didn't wear glasses and walked straight into an extremely sharp metal object that was protruding at eye level. It just missed penetrating my left eye by a quarter inch. The horizontal injury on the ridge of my cheekbone was jagged and required about fifteen stitches. But because the plastic surgeon was an expert at suturing, there is no noticeable scar on my face.

Conversations with others have been the real impetus for broadening my views about living with scars. These intimate discussions reveal complexities about wounds that are physical, emotional, and spiritual.

I've moved from being ignorant to looking and listening with care. I am now a human being, completely present, bearing witness to their retelling and experience.

If admirers want to support you in your work, how might they do so? Are your pieces for sale?

My website is www.lorriefredette.com. Yes, my work is available for purchase as well as commissions. Thank you for your interest and the opportunity to discuss this body of work.

———/———

NOTES

Tauber, Robert. *Basic Surgical Skills: A Manual with Appropriate Exercises.* Philadelphia: W.B. Sunders Company (1956).

———/———

Editor's Note: I have commissioned Fredette for a "scar portrait" of my abdominal scars. She is working from a high-resolution image.

OF SCAR, PALIMPSEST

Heidi Andrea Restrepo Rhodes

Sleeping at the base of my hairline on the back of my neck, it is quiet, and I forget it is there until a lover runs inquisitive lips up my scapula and over the C1 vertebra, towards my ears, and there, an inquiry lands atop my lobes, fetching after the story of this blemish, the distressed skin at my nape, left.

This scar lingers, a rough sketch over fleshly paper, tracing a ghost traversing generations. The mute mouth of a birthmark in the same place as my mother's, and her mother's, and I don't know how many mothers before her, there, below the globe of my skull, rendering its own surplus geographies, concealing furtive histories that waver in my dreams like apparitions, carved out of me by the scalpel to avoid the blight of malignancies on its horizon.

This scar is a mantle sheltering worlds that whisper to me of ancient tales, far away places, and old world sorceries that hex the branches of families or cover them in incantatory armors. Here, in this scrag province, my DNA, ours, has stored the story. Perhaps a war, a firing squad, the hunt of witches. Perhaps a bullet from behind that pierced the cerebellum, cursing our line with the interruption of equilibrium, bestowing on us the disease of vertigo, embedding the dizzy of genocides. Perhaps an amulet burned into the skin, worn into ambiguity over years or centuries of disuse, but which at some time shielded our ancestors from the savage condemnations of a colonial army. Perhaps the coded branding of a hieroglyphic that has secretly awakened our senses in every lifetime, to another possible world and the defiance of gilded patriarchies.

This scar is a trace of things we cannot remember, and the semblance of what is unwritten. The remnant of ferocities and trauma, agonies endured. It is evidence with no record. It is the palimpsest plotted out in the hull: of horrors we survived, or of the invocation of letters that harbor us in sanctuary through the ages.

My finger sketches its boundaries and I remember this small country of wound, the murmuring of rumors from the riddle nevus, its inklings, its estimations, the archive of our old mothers and their treacherous strides.

—/—

"TELL ME ABOUT YOUR SCAR":
NARRATIVE MEDICINE AND THE SCARS OF INTELLIGIBILITY
Sayantani DasGupta

"Tell me about your scar," asks the doctor, sitting on her hands. She is trained in listening, narrative technique. The scar is a doorway, she feels, to the emotional lands housed by the body. And so, she asks.

"Tell me about your scar." She expects to hear stories of fights, times before sobriety, the man who did not love her right, the father who took off his belt too often, the bike accident, the surgery, the botched suicide attempt. Things she can understand, things she can write down and catalog.

"Tell me about your scar." She wants to hear of her patients' bodies, their lives. She wants them to make their scars, bodies, and selves intelligible to her. She wants their scars, in the telling, to become as if transparent.

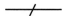

As a faculty member in Columbia University's Master's Program in Narrative Medicine, I have told my students of this technique, this request to hear about scars. I have intoned the phrase the way a priest intones the words of an ancient, holy book; reverently, with passion and belief. In my teaching future doctors, nurses, therapists, and social workers, I have pointed to this question and said, "Go there, there you will follow the footsteps of the righteous, there you will hear, and in that hearing, you will heal the suffering of others."

But I wonder now if that was sheer hubris. The doctor-turned-professor, giddy with her newfound field, convinced that stories are the universal key to unlock the house of medicine. I did not know in those early years that stories can also be dangerous, untellable, unhearable, unsafe.

Writer Iris Murdoch once said, "a novel must be a house fit for free characters to live in."[1] Similarly, in the words of Alice Munro, "a story is not like a road to follow . . . it's more like a house. You go inside and stay there for a while . . . discovering . . . how the world outside is altered by being viewed from these windows."[2] These ideas frame the edifice of narrative medicine—that clinicians must be taught, though reading and writing narratives, to enter the story of their patients' suffering. The scar, by this formulation, becomes a doorway to a patient's pain; an entry point, a surface upon which we physicians can knock and knock and knock again.

But can all scars be told of to all listeners? Can demanding to hear about another human being's scar be a violence of a different kind, a voyeurism, a desire for mastery? Can every patient's experience be explained, distilled, understood?

If Iris Murdoch says stories are homes, what about those for whom the story is not a home, those who are un-homed from their very countries, histories, families, and languages? For all of our privileging of stories, I think it behooves us in narrative medicine and other medical humanities fields to listen to the words of theorist Homi Bhabha, who asks, "what kind of narrative can house unfree people? Is the novel also a house where the unhomely can live?"[3]

In the past decade or more of teaching health humanities disciplines, my work has drifted away from the individual experiences of individual bodies and more toward the intersection of narrative, health, and social justice. Part of my thinking has been about how the scars of history, family, community, and nation are writ upon individual bodies. But what do collective scars look like? How do we in health care recognize them, if at all?

An immigrant daughter, I had always heard how whole countries could be cut in two. The British, on being forced to 'Quit India' in 1947 by the nonviolent and the violent alike, decided they could not leave unscarred the land they conquered and ruled for two hundred years. And so, they took their scalpels and divided the country—Hindus here, Muslims there. Creating scars felt for generations, train-fuls of dead caught in the process of crossing the border; their lives ended in-between, neither fully here nor there. These scars ripple through space and time, scars of communal violence, lost homes and neighbors, lost national identities; entire villages lost on the map—communities who for years did not know which side of the scarred land they had at last landed upon—Pakistan or India?

The scars of that time are, then, multigenerational—felt upon the psyches of Indians, Pakistanis, and Bangladeshis even today. They are seen in continuing communal violence—a Hindu girl killed by her family for marrying a Muslim boy, a Hindu village ransacked and burned by Muslim neighbors, a Muslim village destroyed in retaliation—as well as escalating inter-nation aggression between South Asian neighbors. But such scars cannot be pointed to, like the bumpy mid-abdominal mark of a C-section. There is nothing that a health care provider can see, feel, and identify, saying, oh, yes, here it is, here Mother India was cut in two.

In Rwanda, scars were made upon the memories of a people, even as scars were made upon thousands of bodies by machete-wielding neighbors. In Argentina, those scars were made upon the voices of the people by a military regime who 'disappeared' those who spoke of freedom too loud. In Iraq and Afghanistan, those scars are still being made upon a people by a foreign army who believes they are there to help, whose government has told them they are there to heal.

Who listens to those scars? Those scars along lands: a wall through Berlin, a fence around a Palestinian village, a borderland of patrols, guns and wire between the U.S. and Mexico? What about those scars that cannot be put into language at all? The Deaf children not allowed to go to school to learn sign because oralists like Alexander Graham Bell thought that deaf people marrying each other might create a "deaf variety of the human race"?[4] What about the "lost generation" of Australian Aboriginal or Native American children forcibly taken from their families and schooled in English-only boarding schools with the hopes of wiping out their identities, languages, and ethnic communities?

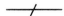

Can all scars be told of? Can all scars be seen? Can all scars be heard?

Maybe we in narrative medicine had it wrong all along. In asking "tell me about your scar" we are surely privileging the individual body, continuing medicine's habit of considering people and their diseases out the context of their families, cultures, communities, and histories. Rather than acting from a position of what Jonathan Metzl has called structural competence (which takes the aforementioned contexts into question), are we, in our focus on scars, keeping medicine myopic?

Is there a way to listen, then, for scars both individual and collective, for pain both recent and long-ago? Can clinicians listen to all those stories of pain—homely and unhomely, tell-able and silenced, personal and communal? Or perhaps that sort of all-encompassing listening and understanding isn't the physician or nurse's job at all. This limit to the clinician's ability to 'know all' through story is akin to the quality I have elsewhere called 'narrative humility.'[5] Stories are critical to medical relationships, yes, but we cannot reify them. As clinicians, we must recognize the limits of stories, and in doing so, recognize our own limits.

The best piece of advice I can give to my students about their ability to see, hear, and comprehend the scars of their patients was given to me a number of years ago by a medical student of mine. Although few colleagues and teachers knew of her illness, this doctor-in-training also

had multiple sclerosis, and so juggled the demands of her education with
the physical and psychic 'scars' of MS. In my narrative medicine class,
she wrote a most moving essay with ultimately this piece of advice for her
fellow doctors about listening: "Try to understand. Realize that you will
never understand. Try anyway."[6]

We all carry scars. Some are visible, some are not; some are personal,
some are shared with others. And perhaps what the very best listeners do
is to approach everyone with that knowledge, but without the expectation
that the scarred will be able, or willing, to tell us 'all', to make us
'understand.' Instead, we keep trying to understand, realize we will never
understand, but continue to try anyway.

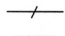

NOTES

1. Murdoch, 271.
2. Munro, 8.
3. Bhabha, 142.
4. Galludet University Archives.
5. DasGupta 2008, 2013.
6. Sebastian, 229.

BIBLIOGRAPHY

Bhabha, Homi. "The World and the Home." *Social Text 31/32* (1992):
    141–153.
DasGupta, Sayantani. "Narrative Humility." *The Lancet* 371, Issue 9617
    (March 2008): 980–981.
_____. *Narrative Humility*. TEDx Sarah Lawrence. April 2012, Bronxville,
    NY. http://tedxtalks.ted.com/video/Narrative-Humility-Sayantani-
    Da;search%3Atag%3A%22tedxslc%22 (accessed May 31, 2014).
Galludet University Archives. "A Deaf Variety of the Human Race." https://
    my.gallaudet.edu/bbcswebdav/institution/Deaf%20Eyes%20Exhibit/
    Language-05humanrace.htm (accessed May 31, 2014).
Metzl, Jonathan. "Structural Competency." *American Quarterly* 64, no. 2
    (June 2012): 213–218.
Murdoch, Iris. "The Sublime and Beautiful Revisited." *The Yale Review* 49
    (Winter 1959): 247–277.
Munro, Alice. *Selected Stories*. New York, NY: Vintage Books, 1997.
Sebastian, C. "My body, My Self." In *Stories of Illness and Healing: Women
    Write their Bodies*, edited by Sayantani DasGupta and Marsha Hurst.
    Kent, OH: Kent State University Press, 2007.

IN THE GAPS

Lanita Rippere

I have scars on the lateral sides of each of my breasts. At 66 years of age, they are not much of a concern to me. I am a married woman whose husband isn't bothered in the least bit by my scars. And in the event of widowhood, I would not be interested in another husband.

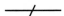

The smaller scar on the left side came from a breast biopsy at age forty. I hardly gave the slice that preceded it a thought, as its formation coincided with the new discovery of my only child, a daughter I had given up for adoption when I was sixteen. At the time of the biopsy, I had just gotten a call from her adopted parents who had searched for me for several years.

Two days after my biopsy, I was to leave my home in California for Tampa to meet my daughter. I was so excited and scared about meeting Teresa and her parents for the first time that I gave no thought to the biopsy. In fact, while I was getting prepped for the minor surgery, I shared my thrilling news with the beautiful young nurse attending me and she burst into tears. She was also adopted and wanted to find her birth mother. Later on, with the help of my dear Jim Taylor, Teresa's dad, we did help that nurse with her endeavor and it turned out very well for her. Together, Jim and I have helped several young women find their birth parents, and it does not always have a happy ending.

I have been incredibly blessed with my daughter Teresa's adopted parents and with finding Teresa simply because the Taylors are incredibly special people. They have a huge capacity for love and have made me a part of their family. I am clear about Teresa being their daughter and not mine, although Teresa and I have a close relationship. She bonded with them as a baby and I could never change that, nor would I ever attempt it.

The large scar on my right breast came from breast cancer five years later at age forty-five. I discovered it on my own in the shower. I'd had a mammogram only two months earlier and the lump was missed. That is why self-examination and body awareness are so critical. I'd had breast implants since my early thirties and now I had to decide to get rid of them. Really not much of a decision. I have never replaced them and only miss them sometimes when I wear a strapless dress. I was treated in California, and I will always be so grateful that I was in such a progressive state. I am alive to share this story twenty-one years later. The scar has diminished to a thin white line now, and I wear it proudly.

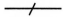

When you have breast cancer, you think a lot about dying. Possible death is always difficult to face, but knowing that my daughter is happy and safe made a huge difference. That gratitude took much of my fear away and helped me to stay positive.

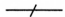

I am grateful I am alive to tell the story of my scars. It is a story that is like many important periods of our lives, which become about more than one big thing happening simultaneously, forcing us to see life's tragedy and beauty all at once. My scars proclaim that sometimes when illness and fear and sorrow carve something out of us, the gap they leave behind can be filled up with love.

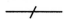

IMAGES AND COMMENTARY
David Jay

"It's not the scars that I am interested in. The scars are merely markers that something has happened. It is the effect of this event on the individual and its reflection in the viewer that I am interested in."

DAVID JAY

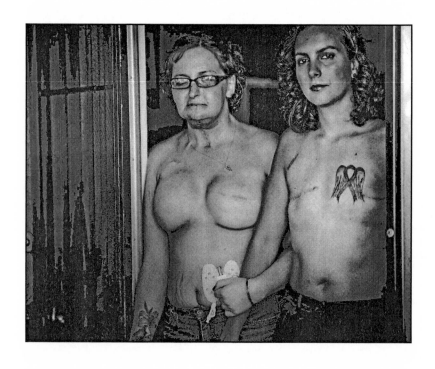

"As a man, I am moved by the quiet struggle of those I see around me. As a photographer, I am implored to share visually what I have seen . . . shedding light on areas dimly lit, trying to articulate in a picture what I feel in my heart. It is my hope these images encourage honest introspection, and serve to illuminate the deep, unspoken bond between us all."

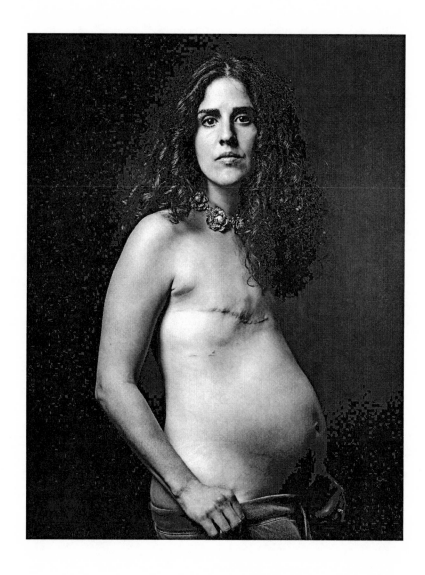

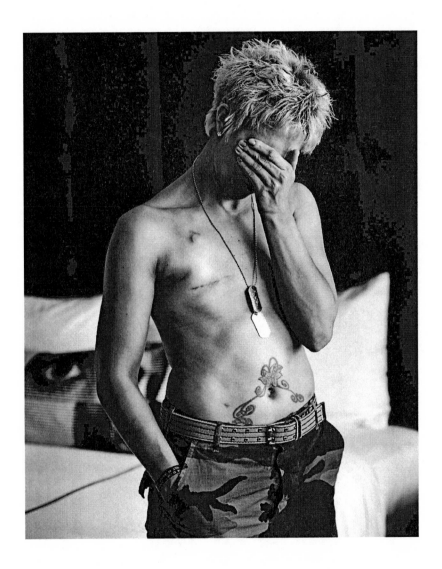

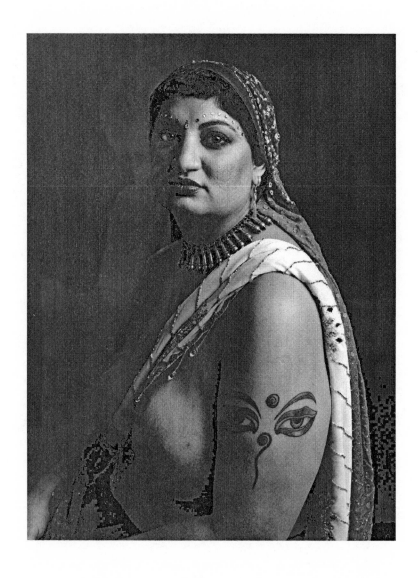

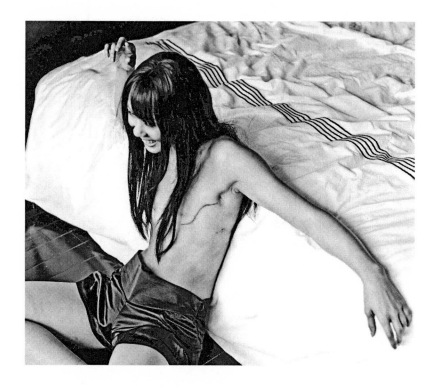

"Ultimately, *The Unknown Soldier* is not about war; its deeper message is one of humanity. Its images transcending the politics, race, religion, greed and fear that drove us here . . . illuminating the scars that unite us all. Perhaps it is about peace."

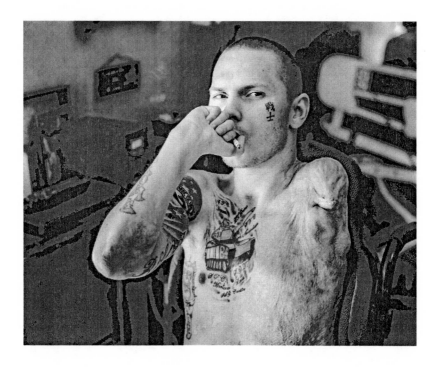

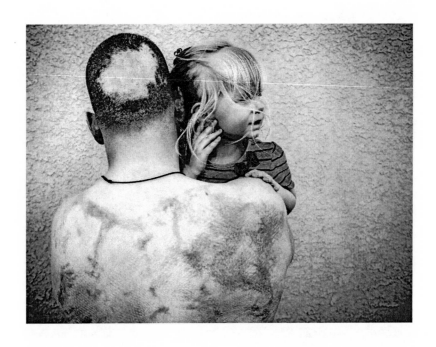

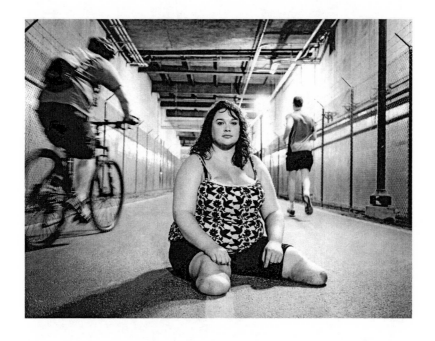

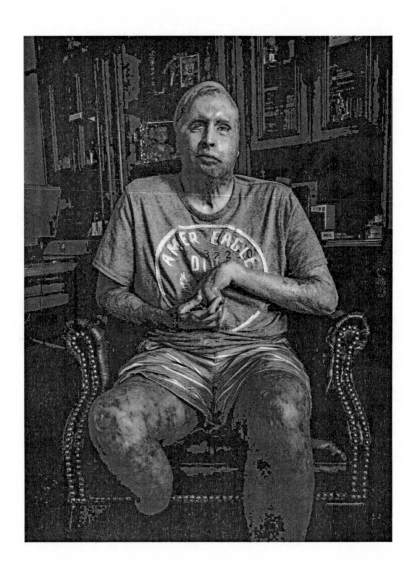

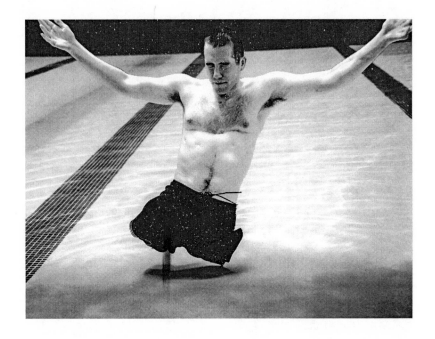

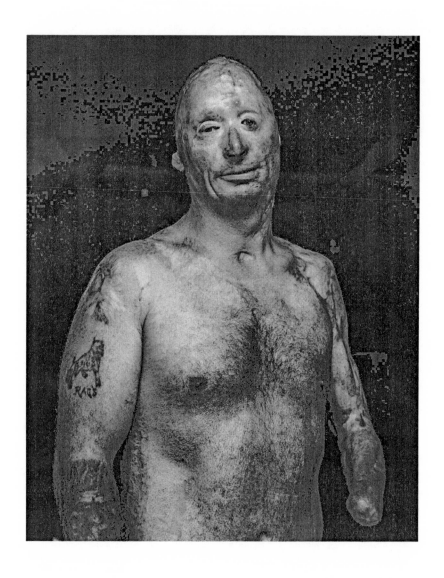

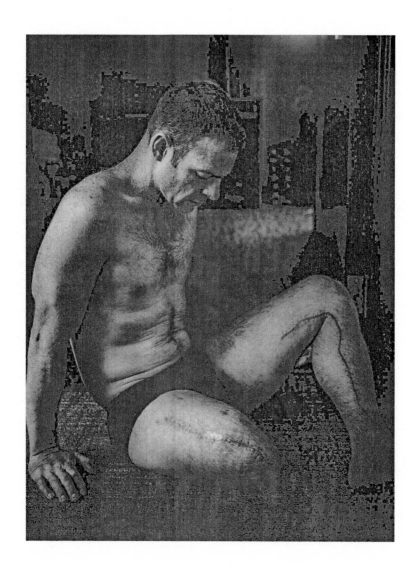

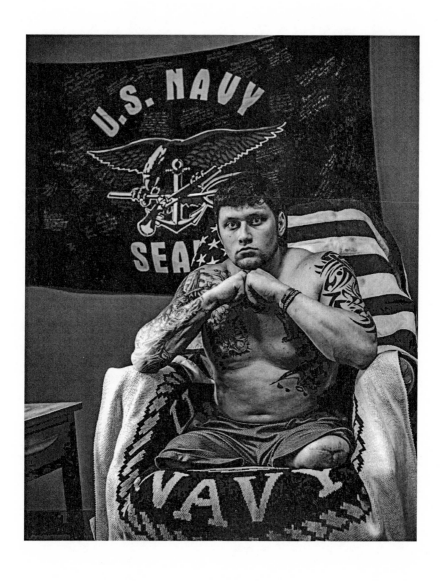

"Still, through all of this there is Beauty. Soul. Courage. These are the things which cannot be taken away."

Images © David Jay Photography

THE CORPSMAN

Jeffrey Paolano

The round enters above my wrist, tumbling its way up my forearm, converting the muscle to milled meat. The ball exits above my elbow although I do not feel it. Corroborating evidence is the hole in my triceps and the sleeve of my blouse.

I see it although there is no sensation, no pain. The arm is numb, hanging limp, the blood now pours down over my flaccid limb.

My right hand still grips my piece. I can still fire, still fight, still make a contribution, still support my squad. I am not out of it yet.

My mind bathes everything I see in crimson.

The world has never before appeared to me blood red as it does now. I marvel at this, examining the strange sight. I try to see past the rufous, see again the green, yellow, and brown, but the bloody red permeates all.

Crapman reaches up, grabs at my K belt and tries to pull me down. I look down at him with languid curiosity. His lips stretch wide as they scream a word repeatedly. "Corpsman, Corpsman," the meaning slowly emerging from the miasma so that now I look about in wonder. *Who is wounded? Who requires assistance? Whose life or limb is in danger?*

With frightening ferocity the Corpsman tackles me, knocking me to the ground. His body shields mine from additional harm as he pulls my combat bandage from the rubber band encircling my helmet. He sprinkles antiseptic powder on my arm, wraps the bandage about the hole, and retrieves my morphine vial, which he rubs between his hands before ferociously slamming it into my thigh.

His features are blurry to me, bathed in crimson as they are. I cannot make him out, could not identify him in a lineup, and would not know him at a picnic. This will not do, I must know his facial contours.

He pulls me up by my right arm, slings me over his shoulder and trots to the evac Huey. He flips me deftly onto the chopper deck.

The empty morphine vial is secured to my blouse collar by its needle.

I stare intently at his face, forcing myself to see through the cerise, to sear his countenance onto my memory so that I may never forget him.

This man risks his life to save mine. The Corpsman will repeatedly risk his life this day as he has done on previous days and intends to do on future days.

I escalate the pressure on my mind forcing a clearing away of the red fog. I am rewarded with a dimming of the crimson and the emerging definition of his visage. The picture is almost clear. I nearly have a grip on his mien when of a sudden his right eye disappears, replaced by a bloody, gooey, pulsating mass. His head is blown back, and drags the remainder of him with it. I see only his body flying backwards. With the bird lifting, the deck edge extinguishes my sight line.

I see, hear, feel no more, blackness envelopes me. My will to observe weakens, overwhelmed by the drug, the shock.

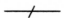

Sliding onto the leather seat, a slide I'd made a thousand times, I raise my hand to attract the barman.

"Jameson neat, thanks." I give a glance up and down the bar to ascertain target density, then swing around for a view of the whole room.

My left hand remains nestled in my lap only to be raised and revealed in the face of the greatest necessity. The Navy saved the arm and the hand at my insistence in opposition to the doctor's better judgment. The doctor felt a better arm and hand could be created through amputation and prosthetics. To honor my wishes, they removed the ruined tissue, leaving three gouges beneath my skin running the length of the forearm from wrist to elbow. The hand is permanently configured with the fingers and thumb in touch. There is no ability to manipulate the fingers or thumb. The wrist is immobile, frozen in place. Behind the elbow there is a concave pocket under the skin created by the absence of muscle and ligament. So much of the muscle tissue was destroyed that the appearance is off-putting, but it is safe behind the bar where no one can see it.

I take a pull on the liquor that I already know will be the cause for my blackout around midnight. Without the depressing effect of this drug, sleep would be unattainable for me.

Just behind my eyes, the memory of the Corpsman persists, preventing sleep, inducing alcohol consumption, fueling emotional outbursts.

Together these factors have prohibited the formation of strong family ties, either with my wife or my children. They have underwritten an irascible demeanor at work, irritating to my colleagues but a decided contributor to my success.

At times my fantastical historical rehash is such that I actually blame the Corpsman, in my replications, for surrendering his life in exchange for mine.

I find I cannot forgive the Corpsman for the slur he has bequeathed to me. Further, I cannot forgive myself for having failed to imprint his face in my memory. As a result I am unable to pay due homage to him, which eats away at me, eviscerating what character I should be hauling along life's way.

The effect is a constant polluting of my spirit. I imagine the foul, bitter taste. I am compelled to retch into my mouth unexpectedly. I wash away the bile with water but the acidity remains.

In this manner I have stumbled through life these many years.

I have prospered financially through the expediency of discovering the ease with which money may be acquired more than any other factor. The only effect is an increase in disdain in which I hold those who are unable to realize this modest goal.

The horizon is bleak. It is as though I look out upon the heaths, uniform in their composition, unremarkable in their verdure and lacking in sustenance. There is no appeal in such a future, no reward awaits me. No realization in exchange for a lifetime of striving.

My space is on the third floor of the parking deck with easy access to the elevator that conveys me to the floor on which my office is located. Without reason, I turn and walk down the slanted exit decks until I reach the ground floor.

I deceive myself by thinking my intention is to retrieve a cup of coffee at the shop on the corner. However, I neither regularly drink coffee nor need to obtain my own. My secretary would provide the beverage in a porcelain cup upon my request.

No, this is something else. There is meaning here, purpose. I am meant to make this pilgrimage, meant to pursue this deviation, meant to discover a new path.

On the street, a girl sits on the curb with her feet in the gutter. She appears to be sleeping, nodding off really; a doze would be more accurate. Possibly she's in the throes of a substance-induced stupor. In any event, her circumstance is precarious. She appears near dead, likely having been on the street for some time. Her boils, pocks, and tattered clothes suggest the ravages of her life.

The building employs a private security force and one of their number closes just now. Just as I notice her, just as I approach her, just as I appear on this spot. *Do I feel the Corpsman's breath? Is he speaking to me?*

I address the security man. "Good morning, this lady appears to be in distress," nodding towards the woman with as sincere an expression as I am able to muster.

The security man looks at me in a quizzical manner. He may not recognize me, but he recognizes the clothes, the brief case, and knows to be polite and amenable. Failing to treat a suit just right could result in a lot of unnecessary trouble.

"Sir, I was just thinking the same thing, that possibly it would be fortunate if I got her inside and notified the authorities. They would know best where she could get the assistance she requires," he said, smiling broadly, seemingly confident there was nothing in his monolog a suit could find offensive.

I look at the security man, trying my damnedest to discern his sincerity. *Would he in truth see to her needs? Did he have her welfare foremost, or was he positing for my benefit and would cast her aside at his earliest convenience?*

Peeling from my roll I hand over the bills saying to him, "I want this woman cared for, and I believe you do, too. Take this money and help her. Here is my card, let me know what has happened to her and what else I can do to help her," I try my best to contrive an expression that conveys I am in earnest and believe that he is too.

I'm enlightened. I experience a substantial sense.

He looks down at the money and the card as he grasps them; more than a week's pay at his ten dollar an hour rate. *Here are clothes for the kids, something for his wife, the payment of overdue bills. No one hands money out to assist him, but this druggie on the street gets rewarded.*

The machinations are unfathomable.

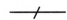

Editor's Note: "The Corpsman" was originally published on July 17, 2014 in *O-Dark-Thirty*, the literary journal of the Veterans Writing Project. The VWP is a 501(c)(3) non-profit based in Washington, DC that provides no-cost writing seminars and workshops for veterans, service members, and military family members. Visit *O-Dark-Thirty* at http://veteranswriting.org.

Where the Bodies Are Kept

Bennett Battle

For now, the smell is only the locker room. It is vaguely masculine and malodorous, but not quite the remembered stench of my high school gym class. Not the musty, heavy odor of pubescent boys peeling sweat-soaked jerseys from hairless torsos, wafting their collected scent into the stagnant air to be trapped by the white ceiling tiles above.

What were those tiles made of anyway? The ones filling the spaces between the long rectangular fluorescent lights that seemed to hum for eternity overhead. With their nubbined lunar surfaces, occasionally darkly ringed and sagging with liquid fullness from some unseen leak, threatening to burst at any moment and release, wet and crumbling, onto unsuspecting victims below.

The smell, instead, contains no hint of what lies beyond the locker room doors. Where the bodies are kept. We are preparing, my classmates and I, changing into our bright blue scrubs before we will enter the gross anatomy lab for the very first time.

I am bare-chested momentarily, reaching to shift my backpack inside my locker before putting on my scrub top. A classmate approaches me and sticks his hand out to my right, so that it is inches away from my ribs. It hovers there for a few moments, awkwardly awaiting my reciprocal grasp, but I cannot reach for it just yet. Since I have now turned my head to look at his hand, the strap of my backpack keeps missing the hook I am blindly trying to lasso.

"I'm Brian," says the man attached to the hand. Just as I finally feel the backpack's weight successfully transferred to the hook and turn to shake his hand the moment has passed and he has withdrawn it, brushing his shoulder length black hair behind his ear.

"I'm one of your gross lab partners," he continues, seemingly unconcerned by the handshake snafu. "I checked the list before I got here. It's posted outside in the hall. Easy to miss. I'm sure most people missed it."

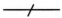

Brian is older than me by at least ten years. I can see now that the black hair is actually streaked with more than a few grays along the sides of his head so that they give the impression of fenders curling above his ears. His ears are pierced. Silver hoops hug tightly against each lobe.

"I'm Bennett," I tell him and put on my scrub top.

He talks loudly enough, but someone is shouting behind me and a locker slams, causing me to miss his next few words.

"E. M. T." he slowly enunciates each letter after I give him a confused look. "The guys on the ambulance, you know? That's what I did before medical school. Anyway I'm telling you this because a lot of people are nervous. That's cool I get it. Spooky. Whatever. People handle stressful situations in different ways. Nothing wrong with that."

"Uh, yeah," I offer weakly. We are now both fully dressed in identical blue outfits. Most of the locker room has cleared. I can see a little inside the lab each time the door swings open as another classmate passes through. I start to lean that way, hoping to encourage Brian to move toward the door. "Maybe we should . . ."

"I just want to let you know," he says, extending his right hand again, only this time so that it presses firmly against my chest, halting my progress before I have gained any momentum. "I've been around a lot of dead bodies so if you feel a little freaked out when we get in there it's totally cool. I've got this. I know I should probably be saying this to the girls in the group, but I haven't seen them yet so I wanted to tell you. I can take the lead on most of this stuff."

"OK. Thanks," I tell him. I haven't really thought about today that much. We've been in school for six weeks, stuck in a giant auditorium listening to countless lectures, so today really only seemed like a chance to actually do something. Even if that something meant cutting open a cadaver. I'd never stopped to think about what it would be like actually seeing that cadaver for the first time.

"Good, bro," Brian says, removing his hand from my chest. "Let's try to get in there before the girls do."

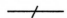

The smell crescendos immediately as I cross the threshold of the lab. Formaldehyde suffuses my first breath, so thick it seems to press against my lips, attempting to pry them open so that it can embalm the inside of my mouth. I feel slightly woozy with this new and powerful fragrance that over the next six months will come to permeate my entire existence. It will creep into the soles of my shoes, coat my hair, inhabit the spaces beneath my fingernails so that no amount of scrubbing with soap and hot water can ever drive it entirely away. Instinctively, I move a hand toward my face, covering my mouth and nose before emitting a series of staccato coughs. After a short while, I compose myself. The stench lessens or at least my sense of smell deadens enough that I am able to carry on, following Brian who seems to know exactly where in this vast room our cadaver is waiting.

The lab itself is a long and wide space that can be sectioned into smaller rooms using mobile partitions that hang from the ceiling and tuck neatly inside the walls while not in use. The concrete floor is smooth with drains set at regular intervals. Rows and rows of waist-high identical metallic silver boxes, each supported by four rolling legs, fill the lab. Fluorescent lights hum overhead, casting a dull sheen atop the perfectly spaced steel cocoons.

Brian and I arrive at our box. Our partners, two female classmates whom I have seen before in the lecture hall but have never actually met are both standing to one side of the box, patiently waiting like everyone else. Brian and I stand opposite them and wait for word from our instructor.

Everyone is quiet as we take our places. A mixture of reverence and fear, nervousness and expectation seem to fill the room. I have to remind myself to breathe.

"You may begin," comes a disembodied voice from the speakers in the ceiling.

All at once a cacophony of opening metal latches shatters the silence. Brian moves instantly to release the latches that run along the center of our box. I hadn't noticed him put on the pair of translucent latex gloves he now wears. Once undone, the box becomes two halves that are connected by hinges to the table's outside edges. They swing up and outward in a 180-degree arc before meeting again beneath the table where they latch securely out of the way.

A sheet of heavy opaque plastic still covers the cadaver, waiting to be removed. Brian clutches the sheet with both hands and pauses momentarily.

"Everybody ready for this?" he asks, looking first at me and then at our partners across the table. We each nod our approval and he yanks the plastic away.

The cadaver is an older man. Pale and naked, reflecting the electric light from above in a vaguely unreal manner, like a detailed sculpture or porcelain cast.

It could be somebody's grandfather, I think.

My eyes travel the length of the body. Along the wispy hairs that finely dust each leg and thigh. Across the wiry gray pubic mound. Up the bare belly and quickly past the chest to take in the face. Shadowed with stubble. Lips parted ever so slightly as if he is contemplating the words he wants to tell us. Eyelids closed. Head bald except for the space just above the visible ear.

My eyes return to the chest. Along the sternal ridge runs a long white stitching like the laces on a football. The suture material is heavy and must be of the post-mortem variety for it is much too thick to be normal surgical nylon. It has clearly been used for its strength and convenience. No need for multiple layers of finely sewn thread for a wound that will never heal.

The man must have died in an operating room. The large wound suggests a precise surgical incision to expose the rib cage that could then be cracked and separated allowing access to the heart and lungs below. But it had failed. The heavy cord betrays a man who never woke up. A heart that stopped beating. Lungs that collapsed a final time. The instruments spreading the rib cage removed. Flaps of skin hastily tied together with the white rope. A job half finished.

I look at Brian standing to my left. He is colorless. Where moments before his face and lips were flushed pink there is a pale and cracked surface. A desiccated landscape begging for the return of blood.

He is another cadaver, momentarily reanimated, as if risen from some nearby table to view his fellow dead.

His lips quiver as he stammers something I cannot understand. His words seemingly sucked back inside before they can escape. I look down to where his gloved hands are now trying to grip the edge of the table, struggling for purchase of the slick metallic surface.

I cannot understand why he is so pale. Why he looks so much like the man on our table. Why the clatter of opening boxes and chorus of voices has been replaced by a loudening hum inside my head.

I force myself to refocus on the table, staring at the man's chest, at what now looks like shoelaces holding him together. I think about the scar that never formed. What I have learned in the lecture hall about millions of fibroblasts linking, piling into microscopic mounds, healing bridges that become one continuous visible scar. But there is none of that before me. Just the bare edges of cut skin. Two ends of cold meat joined to keep everything inside the man from spilling out.

I look back to where Brian stood, but he is no longer there. A small crowd has gathered and I notice him lying on the concrete floor. I feel cold, frozen in place, able only to turn my head toward him. I can see his lips part, words beginning to form. But the words are lost.

It is all too much now. The humming has transformed into an almost deafeningly shrill ring, drowning out everything. I crane my neck to look at the gathering light above as it washes over me and all is brilliant red and blue and purple lakes, congealing into a singular darkness until suddenly there is silence.

———/———

THE HAIRIEST PATIENT:
AN INTERVIEW WITH BRIAN BURTON
Friday, September 5, 2014

in Little Rock, Arkansas by Erin Wood

In November 2013, Dr. Brian Burton, an ObGyn with The Women's Clinic, P.A. in Little Rock, Arkansas, received an unusual call. Because of Burton's expertise in minimally invasive gynecological surgery, the Little Rock Zoo thought him an ideal candidate to perform a laparoscopic surgery on Chiquita, a 44-year-old female orangutan.

Members of the Zoo staff noticed that Chiquita's abdomen was swollen, and it was believed that a previously drained fluid-filled cyst on her ovary had returned. Rather than drain the cyst again, they were seeking a more permanent solution.

Chiquita was born in 1969 at the Toledo Zoo. She lived at the Cleveland Metroparks Zoo before making her home at the Little Rock Zoo in 2006. Chiquita resides with Rok, a 28-year-old male orangutan who had been living at the Zoo since 1988.

Informed consent. How does this differ in animal versus human?

Interestingly, Chiquita has a caregiver, the Zoo vet Dr. Kim Rainwater, who is in charge of her healthcare. Dr. Rainwater and I had discussed different scenarios . . . what should we do if this or that happens. So Chiquita didn't have informed consent, but her caregiver did for sure!

There were nineteen people on Chiquita's surgical team. How does this compare with an operating room in which a human is going under the knife?

This situation was unique in that we had to take an entire operating room to the Zoo. So the nineteen people weren't just members of the surgical team. For example, Stryker donated a whole laparoscopic suite, so their people wouldn't normally be there because the suite would already be in place in a typical OR, but in this unusual case, they sent two people to run all the cameras and monitors.

The other thing with Chiquita is that there wasn't an entire operating room full of stuff at our disposal. Whereas in a normal OR you just deal with issues as they come at you, we had to anticipate complications in advance and be ready for them beforehand. In a typical surgery, you always need a way out of what you're doing. We had to do more forward thinking because there was no out. There was no backup plan.

The patient positioning was different, too. Chiquita's arms were much longer than human arms, so instead of putting her arms at her sides like we normally would, her arms were placed on top of her legs.

I think one of the burning questions we all have for you is: did you help shave Chiquita?

I actually did shave her belly! I don't normally shave patients, but I did shave her belly because I thought it would be kind of fun. So as soon as I shaved her belly and did an exam on her abdomen, I realized the issue wasn't a cyst after all, it was an incarcerated umbilical hernia.

It created an emergency situation because that was not the surgery we were prepared to do. Things changed quickly and we had to call an outside doctor. General surgeon Eric Paul knew I was going to the OR with Chiquita that day. I called him, and when he answered, his first words were, *Tell me you need me at the Zoo*. I said, *I need you at the Zoo*. And he said, *See you in 10 minutes*. He had been jealous that I was getting to do the surgery anyway. So he came quickly and repaired her hernia.

Do you remember the first time that you cut skin?

Oh, sure. It was before I went to med school, when I was a scrub tech in Hot Springs [Arkansas]. There was an amputation, and because it is kind of hard to mess it up since you are cutting something off, the surgeon let me make the cut. He drew the lines on her leg and I made the incision. And it was just really different. I'd never cut someone's skin. So the pressure, the friction, the tension. You don't know what to expect.

Then probably the most prominent memory was when I was a fourth year med student, I got to do a C-section as the primary surgeon. That was a big deal. They don't let fourth year med students do C-sections. But they let me do one. I remember how nauseated I was because I was so nervous.

And your first year of med school, you would have had a cadaver, right?

Yep. The skin doesn't move. It has no flexibility. It is just stiff and rigid. Plus you don't have to be nervous if you make a mistake. So it's kind of a different deal.

How would you compare orangutan skin and human skin?

Chiquita's skin was very, very tough. Very thick. And if you think about it, it makes sense. They are used to living in the wild, so if they had thin skin, every little bite, every little scratch could bleed and get infected. So their skin is very thick as a protection for them. It was very different to cut into a hide. It's really hard to cut through it.

There are three main scalpels that we use, and the one I used for this was an 11 blade. It has a really sharp point as opposed to a normal knife that has a curve. The motion I used was almost like a stab.

Was suturing Chiquita different from suturing a typical patient?

We closed her up, sewed her up in a normal fashion, placing a stitch right under the skin. Then we also put other stitches around on her skin where there was not an incision so that if she were going to play with a stitch, she wasn't necessarily going to play with her incision. They were distractions.

As I understand it, one of the primary reasons supporting the decision to do a laparoscopic surgery on Chiquita was that there was some fear that a curious orangutan would pick at her incision and open the door to infection?

Two reasons. One, so she wouldn't mess with her own incision. And two, so that her incision wasn't weak. It needed to be strong enough so that when Rok was . . . having his way with her, it wouldn't open up. Because apparently theirs is a very . . . aggressive interaction.

Rok. What does the name mean to you? What do you think it means to Chiquita?

Rok is big. He is a big, strong orangutan. So you have this image of him that he's very big and powerful. And he's very sexual, right? I mean, like 10 times a day, he mates her.

10 times a day!?

Forcefully. And so there is kind of an expectation that he would be well-endowed.

But I did a pelvic exam on her, and I could only get the tip of one finger inside her vagina. Generally, her vagina would only be the size it needs to be to accommodate him. And that's it. So I didn't see for myself, but the evidence points to the fact that Rok isn't so big.

So basically, Rok is like a sheep in wolf's clothing, as opposed to a wolf in sheep's clothing. He is a big, burly guy with a tiny, little penis.

Are we violating HIPPA?

(Laughs.) I don't think so.

Were you concerned about repairing Chiquita, only to return her to a life of Rok's abuse?

Apparently this is typical for orangutans. Humans consider it abuse, but for orangutans, it's all they know. And she probably has some comfort in knowing that he is committed to her. There must be something positive that she gets out of it.

Let's return to the aftermath of surgery. You had to concern yourself with Chiquita's incision site. Do your human patients usually follow your directions when it comes to dealing with incisions, which will ultimately become scars?

Most of the time. But I put superglue, it's called Dermabond, over the incision. So it's got a layer, a barrier, of glue over it. So unless they pick off all the glue, they can't get to it.

How much of a calculation is it when you cut into someone what kind of scar you will create?

All of my surgeries on women are based around my incision and my scar. All of them. Most women, it doesn't matter what scars you already have, it doesn't matter if you've got stretch marks on your belly, it doesn't matter if you have a big belly or a flat belly. It doesn't matter. Every woman cares about her scar. So my surgeries are minimally invasive to minimize scarring.

Now I am even doing surgeries that are completely and totally through the belly button. I can do a complete hysterectomy through an incision two centimeters long. The whole purpose of this is to minimize scarring.

So you assume from experience that every patient desires to minimize their scars?

It all goes back to my wife, who had a laprascopic appendectomy during her second year of med school. The surgeon didn't hide her incision in her belly button, and it is a horrible scar. It is short. It is a centimeter in length, but it is nasty and it's ugly. She hates it. I hate it. And so I think ever since then, I've always tried to hide the scars.

When you say you hate it too, is that something you all have talked about?

Yeah. I hate it for her. Why would you want to have a scar when you don't need one?

What about Chiquita's scar? Have you seen it? Did it heal well?

So interestingly, I really don't remember where my incisions were on her belly. I don't remember where I put them. Because a scar to Chiquita didn't matter. It was more about what I needed to do. So it took the scar out of the equation. She was probably more interested in the fact that her belly had no hair on it. Equate it to having surgery on your head, and they shaved half of your head and not the whole head. It'd be weird. Shocking.

What does the physiological process of scarring mean to you as a physician, even as a person?

Scarring is very predictable. Well, long term scarring is not. But the healing process of an incision is very predictable. It gets red and gets inflamed. Then it contracts down. So often if you feel a new scar it is kind of hard and sunken in. And then over time it softens back up. I get asked by a lot of patients when it is in that contracted state, they are really upset about their scar, and I tell them to just give it time and it will release back up. And it does. It almost always does.

Have you had patients who have scarred unpredictably?

Yeah. Of course. Probably the most unpredictable are scars that open up and don't heal. Those are the most difficult.

Like with diabetics?

Yeah, but even sometimes healthy women will have that happen who aren't diabetic, who aren't smokers, who aren't obese, who don't have any of the risk factors. But suddenly, it happens. Even though you did everything the same way that you do every time. It happens, and it's horrible.

I've had a couple of patients this has happened to and it is tough. It's hard to explain it to them and they don't understand why it happened and you start doubting yourself and wondering if you did this right. But sometimes the body does unpredictable things.

What is happening with scars inside of the body? There are lot of people, myself included, whose lives and health have been transformed by scars inside the body. So if you are working to prevent the visible scar on the outside of the body, are you also . . .

Cognizant. There is no way to prevent internal scarring. There are certain surgical techniques that you can use to try to minimize it, but you're not going to prevent it.

Have you spoken with Chiquita since the surgery?

We visited her at the Little Rock Zoo and told our three kids about it. Then we went to the Memphis Zoo, and we saw the orangutan there and they were like, *Look, Daddy! It's like the one you operated on.* And of course the people around you hear that and they're looking at you like, *What is this kid talking about?*

So Chiquita's hair has grown back well. For her, I suppose her hair being missing was sort of her version of a scar. I can't imagine being covered in hair and then all of a sudden you go to sleep and wake up *not* covered in hair. I know when I have a beard and I shave my beard, how different my face feels. It feels cold. Or when you get your braces taken off. How slick your teeth feel. I'm thinking that's probably how she felt.

The hair scar! (Laughs.)

Anesthesiologist Dr. Hunjan was quoted by several Arkansas news outlets as having said, "We feel Chiquita gave more back to us than we could ever give to her. It was a humbling experience in love and medicine we will never forget." Did Chiquita teach you any lessons?

I've thought about that, and you know . . . I don't know. I think of it as a really fun experience.

Maybe one thing she taught me was that with her surgery, I couldn't make any mistakes because there was no way out of it. Honestly, I was probably more nervous than with any surgery I've done. I've operated on CEOs, other physicians, colleagues, and it doesn't matter. But I was more nervous about this surgery because it was true life or death. Not that every surgery isn't, but it was perhaps more true of this one.

A Google search reveals a "Chiquita Burton" listed on Facebook and Linkedin. Is there anything that readers should know more about?

Is there really a Chiquita Burton!? (Laughs.)

Do you expect you'll be fielding calls from zoos across the nation, inviting you to perform surgeries on other animals?

I don't know about nationwide, but I've already gotten another call from the Little Rock Zoo. About a [animal species removed for privacy]. She can't get pregnant.

Fertility treatments for a [species name]!?

I don't know if I am interested in that or not. We'll see.

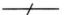

WHAT THEY CAN'T TEACH YOU IN VET SCHOOL
Andrea Razer

The half dollar-sized crater in the cat's caudal abdomen is a window, and I peer through its edges at the inner workings of the feline anatomy. I stand next to the examination table in my veterinary office, shifting my eyes from the cat to its owner, gauging how he might accept the news. Maybe the cat's owner has gone through this before and will take it all in stride. Usually the veterans who have seen this many times will just call and get some antibiotics to pick up instead of presenting the cat to me, so he must not be a veteran. If this is his first time, because of the absolute mystery of the wound's appearance, he will likely puzzle aloud what could have possibly happened. His first question tells me that he lands solidly in the first timer's category. *Hit by a car?* No, it's a cat bite. *Raccoon? Snake bite? Dog bite? Coyote?* No, it's a cat bite. Once I've given the diagnosis aloud, the owner looks again at the crater in the cat, and then looks back at me skeptically. My job is sometimes as much about predicting human response as it is about treating animals.

This is the two thousandth (give or take) cat bite abscess I have seen, but I always explain. . .When a cat bites another cat (which they do with great regularity) bacteria are inoculated under the skin. The initial wound is small, as small as a cat's canine tooth, and usually goes undetected by the owner. If the cat is a rabble rouser, the wound will be on the head or neck— it went into the fight swinging. If the cat is a pacifist, the wound will be on its hindquarters—proof that pacifists need to be very fast runners. The cat will return home following the incident not much the worse for wear, but already seething mounds of anaerobic bacteria are beginning to replicate. The immune system shifts into high gear, throwing masses of neutrophils into the fray to try and contain the problem. Three days later, the cat has a swelling over the original wound, is grumpy, and may be running fever. The abscess could now rupture on its own, erupting like a volcano in a stream of stinking pus, the remnants of dead bacteria and neutrophils. Or the cat and owner may present to their friendly local veterinarian, who will open up the mass swiftly with a large gauge needle or scalpel blade. The abscess is drained and flushed thoroughly. But still, bacteria will remain. Thus, the antibiotics. The owner may turn slightly white or green at the prospect of taking their cat back home with a gaping hole in its body.

Again, they may be skeptical. *Are you sure we can't just close it up?* A few
days of antibiotics are necessary prior to suturing; it will do no good to
close up an infected wound. We send them out the door clutching their
bottle of antibiotics, and with a reminder to keep the cat indoors if it is
summer, lest we get the added bonus of maggot infestation.

A few days later we recheck the cat. A nickel-sized bed of hot pink
granulation tissue is all that is left of the original wound. The owner doesn't
know what to think about the granulation tissue. It looks strange—red
and angry. No, no, I insist, that is happy, wonderful tissue. The owner
casts a dubious eye on it. Again, I explain. Granulation tissue is healing
tissue. Fibroblasts are laying down collagen as quick as they can. In my
mind, fibroblasts are tiny construction workers with little hard hats.
Angiogenesis, the formation of new blood vessels, is happening with
lightening speed, as a multitude of new blood vessels are sprouting
from the vessels present at the edge of the wound. These new vessels
are innumerable and very small, and they are the roads upon which the
fibroblasts travel. It is this proliferation of blood vessels that makes the
tissue appear bright pink or red. Macrophages and neutrophils also travel
these roads, digesting damaged tissue and stray bacteria so the fibroblasts
can do their work. There will be no need to suture this wound, healing is
almost complete. The cat is now meowing incessantly and flinging itself
at the back door every five minutes, so I give the okay to go back outside,
much to the relief of the owner.

If all goes well—as it usually does despite these dramatic and even
disgusting scenes—I might see the cat for a check-up or vaccines a month
later. I brush my hand through the cat's thick fur, finding only the thin
white line of a scar.

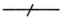

I took Brigita, still attached to her IV line, and placed her in her cat
bed on the floor so my three children could gather round her. I was not
worried about her trying to get up and walk away. She had not stood, or
even moved, in the previous twenty-four hours, and I knew she would
not start then. She purred and brushed her head against the kids' hands
in response to their attention. She was always good with the children. She
was the boss of the other cats and dogs, a dictator, an enforcer. But often I
found my groggy children petting a purring Brigita in the early morning
hours. "I can't get up now, Brigita needs pets," she purred. Her kidneys
were broken, scarred up little things, and they would never get better.
I euthanized her later that morning when she began to have difficulty

breathing, a consequence of IV fluid therapy when the kidneys have stopped functioning. It was the last, best thing I could do for her.

"We're stronger in the places that we've been broken," said Ernest Hemingway. There are many such sayings aren't there? And conventional wisdom to match. That scars are stronger, better somehow, and this is a metaphor for how the psychological wounds life inflicts only improve us. "Well, actually," I might start, pausing momentarily to step up on my soapbox. This does apply to some tissues, such as bone. Healed bone is very strong, though the scar, the callus, is large and lumpy and decidedly unattractive. Scarred skin is sadly inferior to its undamaged counterpart. It lacks sweat glands, and the unidirectional layering of its collagen fibers provides less tensile strength than the crosshatch pattern of the epidermis.

And then there are the kidneys. The problem with kidneys is that as they are damaged and as they scar as a consequence of that damage, the scar cells of the kidneys don't actually function like kidney cells should. Luckily, we (as in all mammals) are generally born with much more kidney tissue than we'll ever need. We can scar up a good 75% of these oversized beans with no consequences at all. But when we get into that last bit, well, as they say, "There's the rub."

Cats are prone to this kind of scarring, which results in what we call chronic renal failure (CRF). Their kidneys are damaged very gradually over months or years, for reasons that are often unclear. More and more kidney tissue, more nephrons, are replaced by absolutely useless scar tissue. Like any other scars, they contract and the kidneys become small and misshapen. Now the kidneys are not stronger, they are just broken. Like our Brigita's.

Contrasting Brigita's fatal scars, my most prominent scar is almost incidental, though there were weeks and months when it was the center of my ten-year-old world. It is large and dark pink, and curves like the new moon across my back. A couple of months of intermittent non-antibiotic responsive fevers landed me in Arkansas Children's Hospital. My arms were soon covered with skin tests for every infectious disease under the sun, which the doctors came and read like tea leaves. An enlarged lymph node in my chest was all they had to go on, and when I stubbornly refused to test conclusively positive for anything, it was decided a biopsy was in order. As a child, when adults tell you that you need surgery and it's all going to be fine, you believe them. I had the doll upon which they illustrated all the things that would happen to me. An IV line here, my incision here. I really was okay just continuing to have fevers on a regular basis, but I was willing to go along with things. Of course, the adults don't tell you, "Oh, by the way, it's going to hurt like hell." Which it did.

While the fevers had made me sleepy and complacent, surgery made me angry. I was not happy with anyone or anything, except the daily Arkansas Gazette my parents brought me. I sat in ICU and read my paper and fumed at the rest of the world that had brought me to this wretched state. And the biopsy? Inconclusive. After all of it, they never did end up with a definitive diagnosis. They ended up suspecting I had Histoplasmosis, a fungal disease. But it didn't really matter because after the surgery the fevers stopped. Just like that.

In veterinary medicine it sometimes happens that you perform an exploratory surgery on suspicion of an obstruction, or a mass, or to biopsy. And you find . . . nothing. And sometimes the patient does get better after that, for reasons unknown. This process is technically known as "releasing the bad humours," which certainly calls up medieval notions of the body, but sometimes it works.

So there my scar sits, largely unseen and unnoticed, by me or anyone else. A good example of the vagaries of our immune systems, if nothing else. The ability of our immune system to heal us is something we often take for granted. And yet, it's not something they can teach you in vet school. They can teach you how the immune system works in excruciatingly precise detail. They can give you needle holders, a needle, suture material, have you practice on a layered foam rectangle until you can make a reasonably neat suture line in a reasonable amount of time. You can suture up your little foam rectangle fifty times over, but when you snip those sutures out ten days later, the same incision remains. You can break a rock in two and bandage the two pieces together, but eight weeks later you still have two rocks. This makes no impact on you until the first time a patient decides to imitate a foam rectangle or a rock. You have said and done all the right things and nothing has happened. They can give you all the tools to make healing as likely as possible. But healing itself, it might as well be magic.

———/———

Day in and day out, I treat kidneys, livers, brains, and hearts. Some of them get better and some of them don't. There are days when everything I touch is dying. I pet furry heads and scratch under chins. I say kind words and give all the magic potions at my disposal, and nothing is helping, and I wonder why I didn't become a lawyer or a pharmacist.

Yet a scar seems to me proof that, although it doesn't work in every case, magic exists. *Voila, you are healed!* I took this little length of thread and sewed you back together and now I take the thread away and miraculously you are in one piece again. You had cholangiohepatitis and your liver cells were dying and I treated you with antibiotics and now you are better. Dogs and cats do not seem particularly impressed by this, but that's okay. Because I am. Really impressed. Every time.

WIDE LOCAL EXCISION

Clairese Webb

As a medical student set to graduate in six months, I had grown more self-conscious than the typical patient. I pursued every effort to accept medical advice and to avoid self-diagnosis. So at the conclusion of my annual checkup with my ObGyn, having kept my mouth successfully sealed the majority of the time, the advanced practice nurse casually explained, "You may have a UTI, so I'll give you some Bactrim."

    . . . but I have no symptoms and my urinalysis showed no bacteria or leukocytes?...

"On manual exam your uterus is very tilted to the right."

    . . . what the f%*^?...

"Oh, and I think you should have the BRCA gene test given your family history."

    . . . yes, my cousin was 18 when she was diagnosed with ovarian cancer, but she's my cousin, not an immediate family member . . .

Keeping my criticisms to myself, I eventually interrupted the summary of her findings by asking if she would take a look at what I always considered to be a birthmark. I explained to her that I'd had it forever, but in the past year the borders and color had changed.

In her calm, attempting-to-be professional voice, she replied, "Oh yeah, this looks like vulvar melanoma. I've actually seen a number of young people get melanoma where the sun doesn't shine, and this looks just like what they had. You don't tan, do you? Some girls use tanning beds and don't wear underwear."

First off, I've never used a tanning bed in my life, and second, gross.

I would recommend getting it biopsied by someone in the next six months just to be sure."

In my mind, I was trying to discern whether to worry or mimic the APN's nonchalance. On one hand, vulvar melanoma is very serious, but then she said I could wait up to six months to have it biopsied? I grabbed my phone and frantically looked up vulvar melanoma in my trusty Medscape app, which had until that moment provided me the reliable clinical information I needed for patients. Suddenly, I was the patient. Peering through salt-laced tears, my eyes managed to catch phrases like "one in a million," "medical management experimental," and worse, "5-year survival rate of 40%."

As I drove several hours to my in-laws' house for Christmas, panic circled like an animal and then lay down heavily on my chest. I was dizzy with grief, isolated in my distress. And worse, I was out of town for the holidays rather than in Little Rock where I was going to school, and where I knew doctors who could advise me. I stopped breathing, thinking the curious beast that is sorrow also requires oxygen. It doesn't.

I solemnly walked into my in-law's mudroom and ran into my mother-in-law. I hesitantly told her that I needed to see a dermatologist and asked if she knew one in town. A stupid tear broke my brave façade.

In my cracked, scared, pathetic voice I squeaked, "I may have melanoma . . . down there."

Shedding tears in front of certain people, for me, is almost on par with peeing your pants; if it ever happens, everyone knows you couldn't help it, but still, it's just a little uncomfortable for everyone involved. I ran straight to the nearest bathroom and hid.

My physician father-in-law called me on my cell phone and said he had a dermatologist friend who would be happy to see me that day. I was thankful my father-in-law wasn't actually home; I never wanted to cry in front of another physician; I didn't want to lose my credibility before my career had even commenced.

I spoke briefly with his friend, Dr. L, on the phone before meeting with her.

She explained, "So your father-in-law told me you have a lesion down there, but I suspect he didn't actually see it because . . . he's your father-in-law . . . right?"

"No he did *not* see it! I just said it's a mole whose borders and color have changed."

"Oh okay, well it's probably nothing. I most likely won't even need to perform a biopsy, but just to be sure, I'll take a look at it."

She was reassuring, but at the same time, her laissez faire attitude hinted that she might be thinking I was simply another paranoid, hypochondriac medical student. This notion was why I almost felt victorious when she looked at the lesion and agreed with me that there was something highly suspicious going on.

Four days after the shave biopsy, I returned to school in Little Rock, ready to start another rotation. My husband Zack and I decided to fill up the car with gas before the week started. I had almost forgotten to worry. As fate would have it, the moment my husband left his seat to pump gas and shut the door, I got the call.

In my own medical consultation voice, I greeted Dr. L and cheerfully shared that I was about to leave for another residency interview, and let her know that the biopsy site was healing wonderfully.

I sounded almost too certain that I had a future.

Her response did not share my enthusiasm.

"Well, I had two of my own dermatopathologists look at the tissue sample, and they both agree that the cells are *severely atypical . . .*"

. . . the crackle of time freezing . . .

". . . but because the melanocytes in that area of the body look different than normal skin, they couldn't say for sure that it isn't melanoma."

. . . gas station convenience store grew hazy, reflex tachycardia gradually failed, blood pooled to my stomach . . .

"So we sent the sample to a specialist in Colorado. At the bare minimum, we know the cells are precancerous so you *will need surgery,* we're just not sure how extensive it will be until we get the final reading."

In a single breath, I replied, "Oh okay, well, just let me know when and where I need to have the procedure done. Thank you and have a good day."

I'm still unsure how medical professionals are supposed to react to the news of their potential demise.

The car door opened and shut, and Zack was beside me once again. He took one glance at my still face, and began to sniffle. We can damn and dam our tears, but they always find a way to trickle down and out. It was evident I needn't verbally elaborate on the situation; everyone's a psychic when it comes to bad news. Besides, he was a year behind me in med school and also knew a little more than the average person about what was happening to me. After a second of eternity, Zack's jagged voice sputtered, "I forgot I have to fill the tires, too."

Alone again, I released my guard and allowed my spirit to be crushed under immeasurable weight, if for only for those blessed moments of solitude. My torso hurled down towards the car floor and let the dammed up tears and phlegm pour. Amidst my emotional tantrum, the logical side of my brain piped up in the background, and I heard myself saying aloud, "Stop it! Stop it! You don't even have tissue! You're making a mess!" I suddenly developed a profound understanding of all my psychiatric patients: crazy lives make crazy people.

I called the person I knew could help me best.[1]

"Ann, how do you go on with your life when you're not sure how much longer it's going to last? I mean, I have interviews and rotations to finish.

---

1. For her privacy, I'll refer to her as Ann.

Should I even bother? Then again, how else should I use my time?"

Ann is my closest and dearest friend from medical school. She was supposed to graduate with me, but was diagnosed with lymphoma as our 4th year started. She, too, was alone when a simple cough led to a chest x-ray, then to a CT scan, then to a picture of a 9 cm mass compressing her heart. The half-moons of her smiling eyes no longer have lashes.

"I know that feeling all too well," she calmly shared. "You're going to be fine. You probably caught it early and will just have to get it cut out; but if you need chemo, I'll help you when I finish my treatment, then we'll take a vacation somewhere awesome. We'll call it our 'I'm still alive!' trip."

Until that day, I had never told her that I loved her. I had never told any friend.

It would be two weeks before I heard back from the pathologist in Colorado. Two weeks of fretting, of pondering all my regrets.

In an initial attempt to venture on, I plunged ahead and attended a residency interview in Texas. The early morning flight blessed me with a window seat and a spectacular view of the sunrise. I didn't peer down at any approved electronic devices the entire time in the air. I could not waste another miraculous scene nor ignore the glorious sun.

My interviewer was a recently retired anesthesiologist from the US military. He was blunt, grayed, and sarcastic. His questions were typical. One question in particular I had heard before: "Most medical students have led privileged lives, but some have suffered hardships. Have you experienced any hardships during medical school?"

I so desperately wanted to try my hand at sarcasm and say, "Well, I found out a few days ago I may or may not have a rare and lethal form of cancer. Does that count as hardship?" I hushed my thoughts, convincing myself that the hospital might somehow hold it against me. After all, how could a resident be productive if she is facing chemo in the near future? I can't remember my exact response, but I don't think I convinced him that I was not in fact one of those privileged medical students. Note to self: if I ever find myself interviewing people for residency, never ask a question about personal hardships because they are, in fact, personal and hard.

After the three-day trip, I returned home, and was left, once again, to stew alone in my thoughts for twelve days of eternity. In that time, I documented some of my dance with insanity. Here's a glimpse:

Waiting Day 1.

This sense of fear is so different from anything I've ever thought possible to experience. There are no ghosts or murderers. There's no one thing that would cause me to scream out because I know that no one can possibly help me. There's a constant level of panic in me, and my mind breaks under the pressure. With each crack, the world pauses and I simply don't know what I'm doing anymore or why. I wish I could cry and hide somewhere. There's nowhere to go. Last night I could not sleep because of a sharp pain that concentrated in my lower back. Today a steady choke has developed in my throat. All the while, the terror rises as I think to myself that whatever I have, it's spreading.

Waiting Day 3.

I feel like a character in a Sim's computer game—an empty shell carrying out useless activities. By filling my days with tedious crafts like knitting, making computer mouse pads, sewing old clothes, my mind has been placed on a shelf, and I see myself in the third person. This morning, I couldn't help but return to my body as I stood in the hot shower. During that brief reunion, anxiety overwhelmed me. For the second time in my life, I let myself scream behind my own grasp. The Sims game recommenced as I soon as I exited the bathroom.

Waiting Day 7.

I started knitting a hat and was very disappointed when it turned out my loom was too small. I fleetingly thought the hat would be cute for when I have a little girl—my first glimpse of hope in the last week. Then darkness consumed me again as I cast the project aside with the realization that there may never be a little me.

The day before I would hear back from Colorado, I went to work at a family medicine clinic. After eight hours of taking histories of minor complaints like headache or backache, I had to share with my attending physician that I would be missing the next week for surgery. Of course, he wanted me to elaborate. I didn't cry but my voice revealed my distress. He then shared with me a piece of advice that I will carry with me forever: "You'll get through this, and when you do, it's just going to be one of those things that makes you an even greater doctor."

The next morning, I received a phone call from Dr. L. She said the Colorado team had the same suspicions as her dermatopathologists, and they'd decided to dub my lesion a "complex nevus with severe atypia, suspicious for melanoma." The title does leave an ominous taste in one's mouth, but Dr. L explained that all the bad cells were mostly located superficially, so I would only need to have a wide local excision done, and no lymph node removal was required.

I opted to have the procedure done by a dermatological surgeon named Dr. D. His office building resembled a quaint cottage. The wooden doors breathed open beneath a mustache archway of stacked limestone. As I entered the threshold, a gust of autumn potpourri sighed pleasantly upon my face. The cheerful secretaries sitting adjacent to a Seaworld-worthy aquarium only added to the sensation that I was being welcomed into someone's magical abode. But just like any waiting area, I was awkwardly situated, facing my physician's other appointments. All four had at least thirty-five years on me.

Age apparently strips one of manners drilled into us as youths, such as the lesson, "It's impolite to stare." For a full thirty minutes, they gawked at me. Their curious eyes squinted with wrinkle rays splayed laterally, but this did not bother me as much as the pity line *between* the eyes, dividing two mounds of fleshy, confused concern. I wanted to shout, "Yes, I may have skin cancer, but no, it's not the result of bad choices young people make like tanning beds! There was no choice I made that brought about this result!" Eventually, I found relief from the awkwardness by watching the clown fish tickle his belly while swaying to and fro along the anemone's bloom. The fish lived up to his title, finding small joys.

"Clairese Webb," the young physician's assistant called me into the concealed chambers of the office. I passed along empty rooms, impressed at their minimal and calming decor comparable to the grand and stimulating waiting area. After passing six exam rooms, my footsteps grew heavy, all the while I was thinking, "Why can't I use these nice clean rooms? Why am I leaving the beautiful sunlit trail and following you to the shadowy corner?" It was like walking into a beautiful castle, then learning you actually have to sleep in the broom closet. We finally entered a room that had inspirational posters leaning against rather than hanging on its wall, and while stepping to avoid those floor traps, I also found myself spinning and dodging stainless steel tray tables set up for various procedures. I felt completely disoriented.

In the middle of the room was the executioner's chair, I mean, the patient chair. It was encased in plastic wrap, similar to a dentist's chair, sat upright, and had cold, metal, gynecological stirrups (minus the ornamental sock drapings), branching out both ends.

The PA explained, "We've never had to use this room before, so we've been using it for storage, as you can see." I could feel the furrow between my own eyebrows as I sat down in the torture device, I mean, chair, and placed my legs in the stirrups.

As the PA set up one of the trays, I caught the sound of a Beatles song gently playing on the overhead speaker. I commented to her that it was quite soothing to have music playing. She concurred. Just as she positioned me to start injecting the local anesthetic, the music ceased. The panging silence and bee sting pricks aroused a panicked feeling. The PA noticed this and offered a small dose of Valium. I immediately accepted her kind offer.

I had elected to have the procedure under local anesthetic, thinking my mind was strong enough to withstand the anxiety because as a physician, I already knew exactly what the task entailed. Looking back, knowing precisely what a surgeon is about to do to you may not alleviate your fears, but do quite the opposite. The Valium unfortunately failed to dull my nerves during the cautery, the tugging, the suturing. However, my physician, Dr. D, did attempt small talk the whole time, which made up for the cruel end of my Beatles music. After the procedure, I was given a recommendation for Ibuprofen (Dr. D had obviously never had surgery in his private area!).

Zach asked, "So you up for pancakes? I thought that might cheer you up?" I nodded yes. I barely recall the drive from the office to the restaurant. Sitting in the orange pleathery booth, I muttered in disappointment that the Valium hardly made a difference, and that perhaps my body doesn't metabolize it properly. Then a numbing sensation surrounded my brain and *thunk*, my melon flopped down onto the table, barely missing my pancakes.

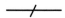

As if I endured a moment in an actual electrocution chair, the physical record of my experience is a lightning bolt scar along my you-know-what. The only downside of this, according to my mother-in-law, is that I'd have to kiss my career as a porn star goodbye, to which I quipped, "Unless my audience has a Harry Potter fetish!" She didn't get it.

As far as my friends and family are concerned, the intimidating clouds of potential terror have rolled away, and the entire ordeal now presents in casual conversation draped with sarcasm instead of fear. I look at their relieved faces and smile, but sometimes it's difficult to chuckle when the chill of another storm stirs along my spine.

Alone with my reflection, I notice my various scars and remember the context of each fall. This most recent one, representing my longest and deepest descent, seems like a marker on a grave, saying "pain and sorrow were here," and I carry it with me every day. Sometimes it tugs and the pricking scares me as a ghost would, but when I feel that sensation, I try to allow it to lead me to thoughts of my strength.

As that wise physician told me, perhaps this will make me a better doctor. Before it, I was pinned beneath the merciless weight of exhaustion. I could not even make the effort to call out a patient's name without first looking at his or her chart. I would only associate name with diagnosis. I hesitantly admit that at least when it comes to doctoring, perhaps I needed this experience.

I am now a doctor who knows where a checkup can lead. Now that I've had this scare, I feel like I'm right there with the patients—*my* patients. Now, I will make every effort to bring them comfort in knowing that no matter where a diagnosis may lead, they won't be alone.

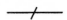

SECTIONS

Jackie Conger

When people think of doctors, for some reason most people's minds jump to the operating room. I guess maybe television has something to do with that. A tense OR with its dimmed lights and moody surgeon is much sexier than a generalist treating sinus infections in a clinic. However it has happened, surgery has definitely become sensationalized in the minds of most of our countrymen. I am no exception. I was always more excited to be shadowing in surgery than in a clinic during my pre-med years. It's an exclusive environment. To be allowed in made me feel somehow that I was on another level, even though the first several times I entered I didn't know much more than the person lying on the table.

During my pre-med years I visited various operating rooms, trying to soak up all of the experience I could. Those times I was only an observer, with the hallmark phrase "Don't touch anything blue" ringing in my ears. No matter what, I was not to touch the field of blue towels that provided a sterile barrier between the patient and all that could go wrong. That changed the summer after my first year of medical school. I was doing a month-long rotation with a family medicine residency that did a high volume of obstetrics. I had chosen to do my rotation there specifically to see as many deliveries as I could. Most family doctors don't do cesarean sections, but in a group that did the same volume as their ObGyn counterparts in town, there were a few who had trained for them, and they were going to let me scrub in.

For the first time, I was going to be decked in blue and allowed up to the table to really be in on the action. I was nervously excited. I went up to the labor and delivery ORs with one of the residents, and he showed me how to scrub, gown, and glove so that I'd be ready. Since it was my first time ever scrubbing, it took me a long time to get gowned up and ready, so I think they had already started the surgery by the time I made it to the table. I don't remember the skin incision, or how they literally cut finger holes in the ab muscles and then the uterus and rip them open. I don't remember the gush of amniotic fluid when the sac was broken, or the doctor reaching a hand down into the belly of that mother to retrieve the cheese-covered head of her new baby. I know all of those things happened—they always happen that way in routine C-sections—but I don't remember any of them.

My memory starts as I was holding the now non-pregnant uterus outside of the abdomen in a towel, so that the doctor could sew it up. It shouldn't have surprised me I suppose, but it struck me that the uterus was warm. I had never seen a living uterus before, and there I was holding one in a towel, with difficulty I might add, while it was still very much attached to its owner. It was like a heavy, slippery, warm loaf of pumpernickel, at least in shape if not appearance. While this was weird to me, it didn't really bother me. I was just very focused on not locking my knees and trying to hold that uterus up.

The room was really hot. Obstetric ORs are usually kept warmer for the babies, and I was covered in blue from head to toe, rebreathing my own warm breath underneath my mask. I asked if it was hot to anyone else, and I think one of the residents agreed that it was. I went back to focusing on my job, standing still and trying not to mess up. I'm not quite sure how the events progressed, but I must have said that I needed to step back, because when I did, I was instantly met by another resident who ripped off my gown and ushered me out of the room. I was swirling in this strange dreamy state where I wasn't quite awake or asleep. I couldn't keep my eyes open and I felt sweaty and unsteady on my feet. I was losing control, and felt like I might drop at any second. In the hallway the resident tried to have me sit on a stool, but I couldn't hold myself up well enough and still felt like I was on the brink of losing consciousness, so he moved me to one of the call rooms and I sank into a recliner. It was a feeling akin to the first effects of opiates or benzodiazepines on a person who is not used to their powers to sap the strength and alertness right out of you. I just sat in the chair, relaxed, but feeling completely exhausted and still unable to pull myself fully back into reality.

It took a few minutes for the dreamy state to wear off, but when it did, embarrassment took its place. I had been in an operating room before, I should have been immune to this! The resident taking care of me asked me if I had eaten—which I hadn't—and as we went to the cafeteria I learned (the rather hard way) that I should have. I was still a bit embarrassed, but I quickly recovered and they all reassured me that this happens to everyone. I heard several of their stories of how the OR had conquered them, and felt at least like I was not the only one who had succumbed. Looking back now, the irony of the situation strikes me. Of all the surgical procedures I could have been in on, it was the one that I would be performing most often in my future career that got the best of me that first time.

I found myself in the OR for C-sections many times in the weeks following that first experience. I was always nervous, whether I had eaten breakfast or not. I was always afraid that I would lose control again, and even though I think my nerves made it questionable a few times, I never did. As I became more experienced, I was allowed to participate more and more, and one day the attending physician told me that none of his residents would be available for the next section, so I would be his first assist. I was very excited to get to have such an active role, but very nervous at the same time. I only had one year of medical school under my belt at that point, and while assisting is just that, it was kind of scary to know that I was not just standing back out of the way where it was safe. The attending I was working with was very nice, and his demeanor and eagerness to teach really put me ease.

Delivering the baby is really the fastest part of a C-section; it usually happens within five minutes of the first cut. It's closing that takes time. After the baby was delivered, he gave me the option of closing the uterus. As a third-year medical student in most teaching hospitals today, your closest contact with the uterus during a C-section is as (sort of) a third assist—wiping and blotting blood so that your resident can see to sew. Seven liters of blood flow to the pregnant uterus every minute through the two large uterine arteries on either side of the organ, both of which lie camouflaged in ligaments. Injuries to the uterine arteries can cause life-threatening hemorrhage, the remedy for which is an emergency hysterectomy. This same attending had told me before of a time this had happened to him when he had attempted to leave the uterus inside the abdomen to close instead of pulling it out like he did normally. He did not realize the hemorrhage until he had closed, and the patient had to be rushed back to the OR and reopened for an emergency hysterectomy. With this knowledge, and a healthy dose of the fear that accompanies inexperience, I quickly declined his offer to suture the uterus without thinking twice about it. I continued to assist as he sewed, and as we made our way progressively out to the surface, layer by layer, he again offered—this time to let me close the skin.

I had heard them say over and over again, the only thing a woman cares about after a C-section (other than her baby of course) is how her scar looks. In the past, incisions were made vertically on the abdomen. If a woman was lucky enough to have avoided stretch marks, that C-section scar might be the only taunting reminder that her body would never be the same again. Yes, this is somewhat silly when named as the price of bringing a child into the world, but as much as we women love our children and would choose them over perfect bodies, there is still a bit of mourning over the pre-baby body that most of us will never get back. Thankfully for C-section moms in the present day, a Phannenstiel incision is used routinely, which is low enough at its position just superior to the pubic symphysis that it is covered by most panties and swim bottoms. However, the size of the scar, even when hidden from public view, still matters a great deal to the woman who is already adjusting to a new self-image.

In the procedure before me, the issue of the "good scar," though still hugely important, was no longer one of life and death, and felt like one I could easily manage, so I agreed to close the skin. As the attending instructed me, he handed me a Keith needle, which is a straight needle, like the kind one would use for sewing cloth. The usual hooked variety required forceps, needle drivers, and a special coordination that I did not possess, but I was confident with the Keith and a single pair of forceps to help grasp the skin. My mother dabbled in sewing when I was a child, and as a result I picked it up. So as I carefully reapproximated the sides of the incision, it felt very natural to me to be sewing this way. I got into my rhythm and slowly and meticulously worked to close the hole we had left in our wake. This woman had never met me before, and probably would have panicked had she realized that she was the first surgical patient of this very green but eager 23-year-old medical student. Thankfully she was distracted in talking to the anesthesiologist, or she might have doubly panicked when the attending asked me if I "had it," and then told me he was leaving. I'm sure I sputtered out something extremely intelligent and confidence inspiring. "Wha . . . what, wait, where are you going?" To which he replied, "Enrico will help you if you need it."

I learned that Enrico, who I had thought was just an old scrub tech who had seen a lot of cases and from that knowledge felt qualified to give me pointers, had actually been an ObGyn in his home country. He was probably approaching 60 at that point, and for various financial reasons had never gotten his license in the US. I finished closing with a bit more humility and the experienced Dr. Enrico by my side, and stepped back from the table feeling very proud of my work, and like a legitimate doctor.

No other hospital I've been to closes C-sections the old-fashioned way—now everyone uses staples. There is a never-ending debate about which method has the best results, least risk of infection, etc., but as no one has yet been able to agree on what is really best; convenience usually wins out, and incisions are stapled. Stapling really does take a fraction of the time, but in a world where I was not rushed, I think I would prefer to close by needle and suture. There is something so much cleaner and neater about suturing. There are no tiny staple holes dotting either side of the long incision, and no trip back for an uncomfortable staple removal.

Mostly I think I just like the feeling of closure—both literally and figuratively—that you get with a simple running stitch. Closing is a way of returning order to that which has been wholly disrupted, which is really what we as surgeons do. It is the gratification I get when seeing the incision I left on a body beginning to transform itself. It is knowing that behind that neat, healing little line I was able to fix something that was out of order, hopefully restoring a function and quality that had been lost, even if only for the time it took to complete a C-section.

I cannot alter what situations lead to scars, but maybe I can help to soften the sting, or add to the joy of their memories. I know that the scars I leave will mean different things to different people, but ultimately my hope is that whatever emotions they call forth will include the memory that the doctor who gave them the scar was a person who cared.

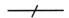

THE WOMEN'S TABLE:
AN INTERVIEW WITH ANDREA ZEKIS

Sunday, September 14, 2014

in Little Rock, Arkansas by Erin Wood

Your surgery. Sex change operation? Sex reassignment surgery? What is the designation you feel most comfortable with?

Gender confirmation surgery. It's a happy term because sex is really attached to the genitals anyway, but there are other types of gender confirmation surgeries that aren't attached to the genitals. We are talking about gender, which is how people relate to the world. I always related to the world as a woman.

As a kid, I knew there was a vagina there. Physically, there was a penis and a scrotum and testicles, but I had a feeling that behind that somehow there was a vagina and the penis was just attached on it. Some people talk about feeling that they have a ghost limb, and I felt like there was a vagina there before, and it was missing.

When puberty came, it was a very traumatic experience because I was feeling things in my body and I'm like, *This is not right. This is not me.* Hair. Deep voice. It was completely scary.

To me, the surgery was eventually became a no-brainer. Something was wrong and I wanted this thing removed. I knew there was a vagina there, but why wasn't there a vagina there? Phantom pussy, my goodness!

When you were younger, were you saying this aloud to anyone?

When I was in my 20s, I wrote it in a diary when I was traveling in Europe. I was away from everyone who knew me as Gary and treated me as Gary. As long as they were in my life, I viewed myself as a guy, but once they went away, and it was just me, in Europe, away from all the things keeping me as Gary, I got to see the person inside myself. And the next day, I wrote in my diary, *The Things I Hate About Myself . . . I hate that I am a woman. I hate that I have a penis.*

In Europe, no one knew me, so it was easy for me to go and buy the clothes of the other gender. But as soon as I went back home, I fell right back in line with the expectations of other people. I was co-dependent.

161

And I didn't know, I mean, how does someone change gender? There was no road map. I didn't meet my first transgender person who just came out and said they were trans until I was thirty. I had no role model. Young people have such an advantage today because there are so many other stories of people doing this that they can identify with and say, *You know what, I can make these changes.* I need to make these changes.

On July 29, 2009, I had dinner with a friend and we started talking about my depression, and we started talking about sexuality, because she knew there were points in my past when I'd been with men. But I said to her, *You know what? It's really about my gender.* And we talked for hours. We closed the place. And that was when things really started moving. But I knew I was going to get the surgery one way or another because I didn't have a penis, I had a vagina, and I wanted my vagina back.

I had tried to make what was on the inside match what was on the outside, and that wasn't working. The only thing that was going to work was to make the outside look like the inside. So I did that.

2012 was a really bad year for you. What were you going through?

The few transgender friends I was talking with prior to my surgery who had gone through it themselves told me that the surgery was basically the cherry on top of the sundae. You've done all this other work—to be yourself, to get the job that accepts the change, to make the friends, and to build up a new life, for me getting a divorce and moving out of my home and losing a lot of the things I had accumulated over the years—and there is the sense that this surgery is the thing that you are going to enjoy the most out of it. The thing that will make it all worthwhile. A few of the people I talked to were like, *It's going to be great. You're going to be so happy. You're going to have this new vagina.* So there's a lot of hope and buildup for that, and it was a hard fall when my case was different.

There is so much focus on the surgery, for so long you are just trying to make a new life and survive so that you can get to the surgery, and no one ever said, *Have you thought about yourself in this whole thing? What this means for you? Have you listened to yourself?* I didn't realize that part until much later.

What did you do to prepare for the surgery?

A lot of big, big things went into this. I found Dr. Marci Bowers in San Mateo, California. I felt like she was someone I could really trust, who had a lot of experience with this surgery. My dad said, *If we're going to do this, let's go to the best.* I'd talked to other people who'd had issues with their surgery, and I just didn't want to risk going through that.

I was seeing a therapist in Little Rock, where I've lived for ten years. I went to Dallas to get the hair removed from my genitals. I wanted to do my recovery with my mom so we'd planned that I would go home to Chicago rather than returning to Little Rock after the surgery. I put all my stuff in storage. Work had given me FMLA leave and I'd accrued vacation pay. My parents covered a third of the surgery and I gave what I could give. I wiped out my savings account. I could have put a down payment on a house or bought a car with that money, but instead I did this. I wasn't buying a Volvo, I was buying a vulva!

So basically, I felt like I was doing everything I needed to do to prepare myself mentally, physically, and financially.

Sounds like your parents were quite supportive.

My mother and I went out shopping one time and I took my clothes off and she looked down and said, *This isn't right. We've got to fix this.* So people were really into the idea that the penis didn't fit with me. Get rid of this part of your body. Remove the penis, remove the genitals, and you'll be like everybody else.

My parents recognized early on that I was still their daughter. And that this was very important to me and they still had to be parents to me. My dad got us a limo to go to the airport in Chicago. We had an extended stay suite. Very nice. They were there with me.

Tell me about the day you went into surgery.

It just so happened it was my thirty-third birthday.

This was a different approach to surgery because normally you would be in a separate room and they would wheel you in there after you'd already been put to sleep. But I just put on my gown and walked right into the room and so I could see everything. It was cold. There was this table that looked like it was covered in eggcrate-type stuff. Like it was soundproof. The legs on the table were movable. I kept thinking, *Oh, my! They are going to stretch my legs really far out and put my legs in straps to keep them in place! They are operating on my crotch!*

I lay down and they were so nice to me and they put me to sleep. I never saw Dr. Bowers come through or anything.

What was it like to wake up?

I guess the surgery was about four hours. I remember thinking, *Oh my gosh, I had the surgery.* The first thing I felt when the pain medication wore off down the line was that my legs had been stretched out to kingdom come. I was so sore in my groin area. After recovery, they wheeled me into my room and there was a curtain between me and another trans woman who had just done the surgery. Dr. Bowers does two surgeries daily, so this woman was in the morning and I was in the afternoon.

The results of my surgery were fantastic. In fact, I remember Dr. Bowers saying I had one of the biggest vaginas she'd done. And I remember thinking, *I didn't just get a vagina, I got like the Cadillac of vaginas!*

Are you still in touch with the woman sharing your room?

I am. She's my surgery sister! Actually our release date from the hospital was on her birthday. So I'd had my birthday and she'd had hers during our stay. It seemed symbolic.

It is worth noting that her case and mine created different financial pictures, which is a good reminder of the range of financial situations of transpeople going through the surgery. She had insurance that paid for the whole thing, so that was a major difference between our experiences. For her, it was like five or six thousand. For me, by the time everything was said and done, plane, lodging, expenses, we're talking about something in the twenty-five or twenty-six thousand dollar range.

What about the few days after the surgery?

I had a catheter in. I was told not to lie on my side. I was all packed up with gauze. There was just a lot of stuff going on down there. After a few days, they told me it was time to walk around. And it was like I had to re-learn how to walk. My legs were all gimpy. I had to re-learn how to pee. And how to hold my pee. I was learning to use all these new muscles. I was constantly living in sweatpants and having to change out sanitary napkins because I couldn't control it. Meanwhile I'm still on Hydrocodone and Vicodin and lots of antibiotics.

What was your healing process like?

There were two wounds. And even with all that hair removal, you want to leave some hair to kind of cover up the v-shaped scars that are in place. Eventually they become hidden through the labia over time, but if you look closely they are there. And they can break open. That actually happened to me a few times. Moving, sleeping on your side. I am a person who usually sleeps on my front, but I had to stop and learn to sleep on my back because it's the only safe way. But you have to press the wounds, and tend them so they don't open up.

Once they remove the packing from us, from the body, and they remove the catheter, it is time to learn to dilate. You are given a dilator that you are supposed to use three or four times a day, constantly trying to shape your vagina. You use a lubricant with it and hold it inside. So after the surgery it's really up to the individual to keep it and maintain it. It's a long healing process to get the vagina to hold its place and you are teaching the vagina where it needs to go. Over time you are dilating less and less.

I was planning to take seven or eight weeks in Chicago to recover from surgery. I was in a wheelchair in the airport back to Chicago. I remember my mom wheeled me in to the women's room, into the big stall, the handicapped stall. And she peed and then she looked at me and said, *Now it's your turn, Andrea.* And then I got on the toilet too, and I peed and she said, *That's my girl.* And to me that was like, one of the most special moments of my life because there was a connection. From mothers to daughters, between mothers and daughters. And I have always wanted to be part of the women's table. You know, you go to a family picnic and there is a table of men and there is a table of women, looking out over the lives that they've built and the worlds that they've built and they talk about things together. Ever since I was a kid I wanted to be at that table. And so in that moment, with my mother in the airport, it was like I was getting an invitation to that table. And that felt really good.

And then we flew back. And once we got back, we had things to work on together as mother and daughter while I was home. We could take my proof of surgery to change my birth certificate and change my social security. We could make those changes together.

So, those were the high points, the cool points. But then things took a turn?

So a few days in, I'm dilating at home a few times a day. I had my own room dressed up for me in the home I grew up in. I was just trying to relax. I'm getting around somewhat, getting around better. And so I'm thinking this is recovery, I'm still achey but I'm getting better. We had my childhood doctor there and he knew everything about what was going on and was ready to help if he needed to, ready to work with Dr. Bowers if necessary.

So a few days in, I'm dilating and I hear this POP! And I was worried—what was this popping noise? Did I stick something in too far? Because these dilators are like six inches long, and you can push things too far.

Then ultimately I go to a Buffalo Wild Wings, you know just out for a family dinner, and I go to the rest room and I look down and I'm like, *What IS that*? I see this dark red bubble on the outside of my vagina. I'm like, *Oh no, oh no, oh no. Something's not right*. I'd only been home a few days and already something's not right. I'm doing everything they told me to do. I'm dilating, using the lubricant they asked me to use. I'm following all the doctor's instructions. And yet, something's happening.

And at the same time I'm getting an abscess on one of my scars and it was getting kind of hard, I was kind of leaky, an area was popping up. So there were lots of scary things suddenly happening. So I went to see my childhood doctor and he drained the abscess and got on antibiotics for that, but the other thing, this dark red bubble that had prolapsed, my childhood doctor was like, *I don't know what that is*. I even sent pictures back to Dr. Bowers and she thought it was weird. She's like, *Maybe it is just some loose tissue so use the dilator and just jam it back up there*. So I'm trying really hard to just jam it back up there and dilate for longer periods to just try to hold it up there. The only thing I can do is to just try to hold it back up.

And then I just realized, the skin is getting looser and thinner and it was just peering out. It was like I had an old man's scrotum coming out of my vagina. And I'm trying to keep it clean and sterile. I'm trying to hold my vagina in my hands while I pee and poop. It got to the point where I gave up on the dilator and was just trying to push it up there with my fingers. And at the same time I'm trying to heal on the outside. So its like, everything is so vulnerable. I'm trying and trying and it's just not working.

I went back into my childhood doctor and he was like, *I don't know what to do with this, and if I were you I'd go back to California*. So less than a month after the surgery, we're flying back.

How did you feel, flying back to San Mateo?

I felt like a failure. I felt like I was broken. It was like, *Why me? Did I do something wrong?* I took most of the fault on myself. This was supposed to be a momentous occasion and instead I'd spent the last twelve days holding my vagina in my hands trying to keep it clean. And I just kept thinking, *This isn't how this is supposed to be. Is this ever going to get fixed?*

And so it was another week in California trying to get this resolved. It was a totally different feeling than the first time we went to California. We were on a mission. We had a smaller room. There was no limo. It was like we were just crawling back. And it was just sad. It was a sad week.

And what happened when you saw your doctor again?

She saw me in her regular gynecological office. She just said, *Oh my dear, I'm so sorry you had to go through this.* She said she hadn't seen anything like my case in years. Another had been a diabetic. So I start thinking *Woah, are there other issues with me? Now am I diabetic? What's wrong with me?* There really wasn't an explanation for what was happening.

With great care and immediacy in order to keep me calm, she removed what had become dead tissue. I focused on a picture on the wall, and didn't feel a thing. By the time I looked down, I had been freed of the tissue that I struggled to save and keep clean, and became repacked with gauze to soak up the blood. She said there was no way to save the skin, but despite the gloom and doom in my mind, she assured me I still would have a good result.

My entire cavity was a skin graft inside. She explained that I would probably just end up having some scar tissue. I didn't know how to feel about that. I was in shock. Scar tissue would have to form in place of the skin and my recovery might be prolonged, but she told me some surgeons don't put in the skin graft—like she did in my case—leaving their patients having to work with scar tissue after surgery. She really tried to help me think not about what I lost and what I've been through, but what I still had and had to look forward to. The hellish twelve day period came to an end and I prepared for a new normal.

Is scar tissue less desirable in some way?

Well it takes a lot longer to heal. Things are a lot more vulnerable. You can have granulated tissue and you'll be bleeding more over a period of time. And then it was like not only would I have these two wounds on the outside, I would also have a scar on the inside that no one could see except me and my gynecologist. But still, a scar.

So, the entire skin graft was removed, and I didn't have it anymore. The entire scrotal skin graft that I'd spent all that time and money getting all the hair removed from and dealing with carefully. It was gone. I didn't have it anymore.

I got packed up with stuff again. And I was constantly bleeding whenever I was dilating. And then I was on pain meds because everything hurt.

So in order to heal, in a way you were having to inflict more pain on yourself through the dilation process?

Right.

And it didn't seem like there was any kind of answer? Were you afraid this might happen again?

Yeah, and so oddly my mom is going through menopause at the same time and trying all these lubricants so I'm trying them, and the next thing I know I have a UTI and I'm in the emergency room. And they are coming at me with the most enormous speculum I've ever seen in my life. My mom was like, *You are not putting that in my daughter.*

But anyway, there's just all this stuff that keeps happening. And it's about that time that we started thinking, huh . . . maybe this could be the lubricant that's causing the problem. But I couldn't dilate without it, so I needed to find something I could work with. I couldn't naturally lubricate myself, but I had to dilate.

And then my time had run out. It was time to go back to Arkansas. I had to get back to work. I had to move. And I wasn't allowed to lift anything so I'm paying for furniture to be moved here and there. I was still in pain and worried. I was still on antibiotics. I had to scramble to find a place to live and then had to move again because the first apartment where I went wasn't safe for me. I was having to carry two rents at one point. And then I'm just not healing and I'm feeling this awful burning feeling every time I used lubricant.

Then I found coconut oil and I didn't seem to have a problem with it, and eventually an all natural product called Sliquid. So then it was pretty clear in my mind that lubricants were the cause of the prolapse. And I realized that I just hadn't been listening to myself.

What do you mean by "listening to myself"?

I'd been listening to everyone else and their advice, but not to myself. I trusted so many other people who didn't know my body instead of listening to my own body. If I'd listened to my own body, maybe I could have prevented the prolapse.

There was a point of acceptance. This is what my body is and this is what I can do with it. I think we all accept some of our limitations, but for me it was accepting that I was going to have a longer recovery. For so long, I was still bleeding. And I realized I needed to take some time back and take care of myself. I didn't have all the good bacteria inside my body so that my vagina could take care of itself like most women do. I had to build that up.

So if you were bleeding all this time, was new scar tissue forming?

Yeah, yeah. There were actually little pieces of skin coming out of me when I dilated. It is almost like raping yourself on a regular basis, just to keep it going. Just to keep it from closing. It made sex completely not attractive at all.

To you, or did you have a sense that it would be unattractive to someone else?

Yes. To me. For two years. Because whenever I did have sex with someone it would cause trauma and it would bleed. It was like I was always on my period. And I'd always wanted to have a period because it was a part of what women go through and I wanted that but then I was like . . . I got more than I bargained for, actually.

So I still felt broken for a long time. I was still on painkillers. I was getting addicted to the painkillers because I didn't want to feel anymore.

How did you go on?

A couple of things changed my life.

One is that we found a lubricant that would work that wasn't coconut oil. My mom and I. Our bodies are so similar that we were both trying them out and comparing notes. So we found the Sliquid. If it wasn't reacting to her it wasn't reacting to me. Having my mother there to talk with about everything made a huge difference. Without her, I'd have been lost. My mother was my saving grace.

And second, I started getting into more activism. Being involved in the community made me stop focusing so much on myself and start thinking about others. I could heal in that respect because I was no longer like, *Woe is me* and, *Look at my broken vagina.* I started thinking, *Maybe I'm okay and I'm on my way to recovery. Maybe I can think outside myself.*

Maybe it is really good for your voice to be out there so that the message you lacked, the one that set up the expectation for the cherry on top and nothing going wrong, might prepare others a little bit for the things that can go wrong?

I'm a lot more pragmatic after the surgery. A lot more realistic. I don't want to jade anyone else and say don't do this, but there was no one else out there like me. I had to make decisions for myself. So maybe that's the preparation or the message I can help with.

The decisions of others are fine but they won't do for me. After the surgery, and discovering the limitations of my body, I decided I wasn't going to do any more surgeries. There are folks out there who have lots of surgeries on their lists . . . *Oh I want to have the nose job or the breast augmentation or the trachea shave* and other stuff like that. But for me, after this, I just realized this was it. I mean, how might my body react to breast implants? My recovery from this surgery was so long, why would I want to do something else to my body? So after the surgery, I think of myself in a completely different way.

And so I have just taken all my inadequacies, the things about myself that I felt were inadequacies, and put them into my work. So I did whatever I could to feel like a complete person and to be able to accept myself as myself. Being an activist, supporting others, it has helped me heal. It has given me the time to feel like I'm okay with me.

You were listed as a Visionary Arkansan 2014 by *Arkansas Times* because of your impact on social justice. You've founded the Arkansas Transgender Equality Coalition. Does this transition into a life of activism take too much of you sometimes?

It's easy to focus on the activism and not on my own body. So I try to remember to rest. I want to rest. I have continued seeing a therapist, who has determined I have PTSD from surgery and that happens to some people. So I'm glad to have someone to talk about it with. And I've kept the same therapist. Some transpeople do the therapy up until the surgery and then after it, the therapist signs off on their letters and they quit going. But I want to go on because I feel like there are so many more ways for me to grow after the surgery. I mean, what is my life like after it? It's not the way I thought it was going to be. It's not all sunshine and lollipops. It's something more real. Something more true to who I was. There was no cookie cutter way to transition. For me it was going to be a different story.

Have you been back to see your doctor?

I went back for a year check up in California. My doctor looked things over and she said, *You know what? It looks fantastic. You have some granulated tissue, but you know what? It looks fantastic. The granulated tissue is to be expected with what you went through.*

How did hearing her words make you feel?

Like I was no longer broken. Like I can move forward. I've found a doctor here in Little Rock who sees me every four months or so, to remove the granulation tissue, and to give me silver nitrate treatments. I've finally stopped bleeding on a regular basis.

I can finally have vaginal intercourse with no problems. But it's taken two years. For so long, it was all inadequacies. I always thought about what I wasn't getting and what I couldn't have. But now I can have something. Finally I can have something.

My scars are a part of me; we have gone through a lot together. I've realized that what others do is not a reality for me. I am not like any other woman. But I guess what I've learned in the end is that I haven't gone through this process just to be like another woman; I've gone through this process just to be myself.

You walk on stilts, which is kind of unusual. Why do you choose that activity?

I started walking on stilts in 2013. I'd had this fear of heights that had kind of eroded with my transition, but I wanted to test it out and see where I could go with it, so I paid $50 and signed up for a class. I wanted to find out what my feelings were.

I went to the class and there were four of us. And I was the first person to walk around without my hand on the wall, which also meant I was the first person to fall. And then the instructor taught us how to fall. And once he taught us how to fall I was like, *Ah! I can do this!* Because once you know how to fall, the fear is gone.

It's the same thing with the surgery stuff . . . If you know how it could be, how things could go wrong, what it might be like, then you don't worry about it as long. See, no one had talked about a prolapse. They had talked about granulation tissue, or open scars, but no one ever talked about what happened to me. No one ever said, *If your hoo-ha pops out, here's how to take care of it.* So when the prolapse happened, when I started to fall, I was terrified.

For me, stilt walking creates a moment to be free. Outside of my own body. You can't think about your everyday activities like what you'll make for dinner. You have to be there. Present. You are constantly moving. Your eyes are forward. You are moving. So it's an opportunity to do something completely different. It's a place I can go that not many other people can go. Its freeing, and it had a big role in my recovery. I think there's a point when you feel broken that you think your life is over, but then all the sudden an opportunity opens up; stilt walking was like that for me. I can go up there and the sky is the limit. There is a life for me after this.

How do you feel about sharing your story publicly?

Even during the time of the surgery, I didn't want to stand out. I was living openly as a trans person in different areas of my life and not in others. I might be open at my job, but then when I would go to temple, I wasn't. In different spaces, I was different people.

One of my activist mentors I look up to explained to me that in the age of the internet there is no such thing as stealth. If you run away from it, you run away from who you are. There are pictures and videos and snippits of you out there and you can either own it or other people are going to own it for you.

I feel like in order to be who I am now, I have to love not only who I am right now, but I have to love the person who I was, even the part of me that was broken.

Do you have any thoughts on what you wish those who haven't gone through this surgery would recognize? Not necessarily trans people planning to go through the surgery, but more broadly what people in general could learn from your personal experience?

There is the writers' notion of *killing your darlings* . . . You have things you really covet, that you really love, which color the entire way you look at things because of this one belief. But you might be losing the whole story because you are trying so desperately to hold on to this one piece of it. I focused so much on getting to surgery, getting through surgery and the aftermath, that I detached myself from how I truly felt about myself and really did not see all the other great qualities and experiences in my life. If you work so hard on this one piece of your life that you want to get fixed, you might be missing the rest of the picture. So maybe getting rid of that one thing that you think is so big might be blinding you to big problems ahead or blessings in disguise. The decisions I made about myself shouldn't define everything about me, they are just one part of a whole person. When putting a vagina on a pedestal, make sure to put your whole self on the pedestal at the same time—and that goes for anyone's major life decisions.

How did the surgery change your view of scars overall?

I grew up thinking that my appendectomy scar showed how brave I was because of the physical things that I'd lived through (severe weight loss, a nearly burst appendix). But these recent scars make me think, *Maybe it is even more brave that I became who I am.*

I decided to be me and to be me wasn't just to be a woman, but to be Andrea Zekis. And who is Andrea Zekis? That is still evolving and I don't want to stop just yet. I have become not so afraid of change anymore. There was one point where I was very afraid of change, but I'm no longer afraid.

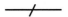

WRITING THE BODY:
A FEMINIST PERSPECTIVE ON SURGICAL SCARS

Melissa Nicolas

I have four visible surgical scars: three purplish dashes and one brownish dot on my abdomen. Since I stopped wearing bikinis in the last millennium, these scars are visible only to my partner, some doctors, and me. My scars are not physically painful, and since they are invisible to almost everyone, I do not think much about them on a daily basis. On my flesh, however, the scars indicate physical trauma: two emergency surgeries—one in my late thirties for a ruptured appendix and another in my early forties for an inflamed gall bladder.

Each of the four scars is within six inches of the others. If you connect the dashes, you would have a messy isosceles triangle with a dot in the middle. These scars are different from some other scars on my body. For example, I have a small scar on my right hand from a deep cut when I was ten-years-old. The scar on my hand does not "speak" to me; I do not attach any specific meaning to it other than I was a bit careless when I was ten. The scars on my abdomen, however, have gotten under my skin, so to speak.[1] *Why are there so many scars in such a small area of my body? Why has my body been etched this way?* I am a scholar of rhetorical and feminist studies, so when I am looking for answers to questions like these, I turn to the areas that I know best. In trying to write my body, I want to look beyond the medical reasons that precipitated these two surgeries and explore how these scars are telling a much more intense story than that of inflamed and burst organs. Using the idea of the somatic mind—that my mind and body are constantly creating and recreating the narrative of my embodied being—I hope to illustrate the incredible power of writing the body.

At the beginning of the twenty-first century there has been much work in the medical field, particularly neuroscience, illustrating how thoughts and feelings interact with the endocrine system to produce hormonal effects in the body.[2] What scientists are proving through empirical experiments is that instead of the mind and body being two discrete and independent systems, they are collaborative partners who together produce physical sensation, thought, and emotion. The mind and body talk to and inform each other; they are interconnected and intertextual. It seems the sciences and humanities have found common ground in exploring the mind/body connection.

To best understand the psychological and emotional climate under which my emergency surgeries took place, some context is in order. The appendectomy took place on a Saturday, the day of the first open house on a home we were trying to sell as a short sale. We had been in the house for a little over a year and suddenly found ourselves underwater with our mortgage. In addition, my partner lost his job and we had a nine-month-old son. We knew we had to get out of the house, even if it meant loosing money, but the stress of our financial and housing situation was taking its toll on me. At the time, I was seeing a therapist, but I was not fully exploring the anger, frustration, and disappointment that were roiling inside me. Additionally, because we had an infant, I was constantly exhausted. I tried and tried to keep a tight lid on my feelings, fearing an emotional explosion if I let anything go.

While my mind tried to control my emotions, my body refused to absorb the pain and anger, and I had the feared explosion—an expulsion, really—but it was not the psychological kind I was expecting. Instead of an emotional breakdown, a piece of my body became so inflamed that it exploded, the lethal juices from my appendix seeping into my system, necessitating a post-operative drain. The thing I most feared—a serious outburst that would hurt someone or something—did indeed happen, but not as I expected. The explosion took place inside of me, and it did hurt, both physically and emotionally. My body had enough negative energy inside that it responded by acting-out. According to psychologist Theodore Sarbin: "[. . .] emotional life is embodied."[3] So at least for Sarbin, it is indeed possible that my excessive negativity became manifest in my body through a literal bursting of one of my organs.

My second emergency surgery happened six years after the appendectomy. This time, the emergency came on a Wednesday while I was on sabbatical. Given the lack of committee assignments, office hours, and piles of grading, all seemed calm in my external world. However, internally, there was chaos, and I was not seeing a therapist. I was recovering from a period of severe stress and loss and while my symptoms seemed under control, I feared they would return or become worse. As before, I was swallowing as much of the fear and anxiety as I could. My gallbladder did not burst the way my appendix did, but by the time I made it to the ER, a biopsy showed my gallbladder was inflamed and on its way to ripping apart. There was a good chance that if left inside me, it would have burst at some point in the near future. Additional information emerged from the surgery, too. Using a scope, the surgeon discovered that my colon was also inflamed and distended. Subsequent testing confirmed that I had an "angry" and "tortuous"[4] colon that might need surgical intervention soon.

My surgical scars, then, signify a series of events that have happened to my actual living, breathing body. The meaning I ascribe to these scars (the remnant of the lived experience) and the body that holds them is constantly under discursive construction.[5] At first, these scars were just that: marks on my skin. But as time has passed, my mind has worked in concert with my body to produce new and fluid meanings about these marks. Kristie Fleckenstein has named this body/mind connection the "somatic mind," acknowledging the intertextuality between the mind and body. According to Fleckenstein, "The concept of the *somatic mind*—mind and body as permeable, intertextual territory that is continually made and remade—offers one means of embodying our discourse and our knowledge without totalizing either. This 'view from somewhere' locates an individual within concrete spatio-temporal contexts."[6]

The "view from somewhere" of the somatic mind allows us to bring the body into discursive existence while simultaneously allowing for the body to hold its own significance in shaping that existence. To argue otherwise— to believe that the body is solely constructed through discourse—is to erase the actual physical body that exists in time and space. In Fleckstein's words, "Embodiment is required for meaning and being."[7] For Fleckenstein, there can be no free-floating meaning; meaning must be anchored in a real, physical body, and, in turn, the body will shape its own meaning through its very existence. Surgical scars—parts of the body where discursive constructions of an event (often, a traumatic event), and the flesh meet— are critical pieces of the intertextual narratives that shape existence.

From a feminist perspective, the concept of the somatic mind participates in Hélène Cixous's call to "write the body." Historically, women have been identified with the body, most obviously in relationship to childbearing. The body, and therefore women in the Western tradition, have had a hard time of it. Plato "disregards" the body[8] while other great Western thinkers, such as Descartes, reason that only the mind needs to exist to prove existence.

As such, when philosophers, scholars, and historians disregard the bodies of women, treating those bodies as curses to be broken rather than as critical parts of being, the body (women) are relegated to an inferior existence.[9] Our contemporary language still holds remnants of these patriarchal attitudes about women's bodies and their bodily functions.

Indeed, "the curse" is used pejoratively to refer to women's menstrual cycles. As Andrea Lunsford reminds us, "the realm of rhetoric has been almost exclusively male not because women were not practicing rhetoric— [. . .]—but because the tradition has never recognized the forms, strategies, and goals used by many women as 'rhetorical.'[10] For women, many of the "forms, strategies, and goals" used in their discursive practices are embodied. In other words, unlike Descartes's privileging of the mind almost to the exclusion of the body, women's rhetoric often situates the body and mind as co-equal.

Cixous illustrates how women have been discursively constructed by the Western tradition as evil, but she presents a way for women to assert their own embodied rhetoric. As an example, she re-reads the myth of Medusa. In "The Laugh of Medusa," Cixous claims that Medusa, in all of her snake-covered glory, is "beautiful and she is laughing."[11] Unlike traditional readings of this myth where Medusa is situated as figure to be feared and killed, Cixous paints Medusa in a completely different light. To take a mythological figure that has been classically associated with death and make her, instead, a symbol of beauty and joy upends the very roots of western history and rhetoric. In the Medusa myth, anyone who looks the Medusa in the eye is turned immediately to stone. While there is nothing in the myth that says women are not equally affected by her death stare, most of the stories we have about Medusa are of men turning to stone after gazing upon her face. What if Medusa's great power was not that men turned to stone when looking at her but rather that men's *fear of looking* at her is what turned them to stone? What if someone were brave enough to look at her straight on without fear? Cixous suggests that looking without fear would reveal a Medusa—a fully embodied gorgeous Medusa—that would bring joy. Perhaps, it is the masculinist *fear* of a righteous babe with mad hair who is fully embodied, powerful, competent, and intelligent that strikes fear into men's hearts, turning them to stone. By marking Medusa as evil, no one has to reconcile her bodily identity and intelligence—she is doomed, both in body and mind, to an evil pantheon because of her body.

———/———

For Cixous, the job of women is to write themselves back into history, like she does with Medusa, through recovering their disregarded bodies: "Woman must write herself: must write about women and bring women into writing, from which they have been driven away as violently as from their bodies—for the same reasons, by the same law, with the same fatal goal. Woman must put herself into the text—as into the world and into history—by her own movement."[12] Cixous calls on women to reclaim their bodies, not only to acknowledge the existence of the flesh but also to discursively celebrate the connection between their sense of self and their bodies. By acknowledging and celebrating the body, women and men can look upon the Medusa without fear and hear her laughing. In effect, by re-reading the Medusa myth, Cixous provides us with a way to read and write the body from a non-patriarchal perspective.

Writing about corporeal scars is another way to write from a different perspective; in dealing with physical scars, we cannot overlook or disvalue their visible, bodily presence on the skin. Even though much of what we say about our scars may be emotional or psychological, the physical scar is always a reminder of the embodied nature of the trauma that led to the scarring. Social psychologist James Pennebaker explores the connections between writing about trauma and emotional health. He theorizes, based on experimental and empirical data, that there is significant therapeutic value in writing about trauma. Indeed, Pennebaker suggests that not only is writing about trauma good for you but also that not writing (or talking) about it can further harm your emotional and physical health: "Holding back and not talking about an upsetting experience is bad in and of itself because of the physiological work of inhibition. A deeper problem is that when individuals inhibit, they fail to translate their thoughts and feelings into language. Without resolving their traumas, they continue to live with them. The health benefits of writing or talking about the traumas, then, are twofold. People reach an understanding of the events and, once that is accomplished, they no longer need to inhibit their talking any further."[13] To not write about scars, therefore, is unhealthful for the somatic mind because it forces a performance of inhibition. Inhibition can force a wedge between the body and mind, keeping the two from constructing a coherent co-narrative about the trauma or event that precipitated the scar. To keep the body and mind apart takes hard mental and, as we are learning, physical work that ultimately depletes both body and mind.

While writing about trauma and its visible reminders (scars) contributes to the healing of the somatic mind, this kind of writing is also an act of writing the body. If the somatic mind does not recognize barriers between the mind and body, then writing about thoughts and feelings (mind) cannot help but influence the body. Pennebaker's work provides some evidence of this process: "[. . .] actively holding back or inhibiting our thoughts and feelings can be hard work. Over time, the work of inhibition gradually undermines the body's defenses. Like other stressors, inhibition can affect immune function, the action of the heart and vascular systems, and even the biochemical workings of the brain and nervous systems. In short, excessive holding back of thoughts, feelings, and behaviors can place people at risk for both major and minor diseases."[14] The body and mind talk to and write each other. Scars are but one piece of evidence about this process. A scar from surgery is the visible manifestation (i.e. embodiment) of a lived event and all of its subsequent emotional and psychological consequences.

Building on the premise that the mind and the body have an intertextual relationship, another avenue for analyzing scars emerges. In an intertextual relationship, meaning is made in the "inter" between the texts, through the texts, around the texts; texts speak to each other and respond to each other and create and re-create themselves. Intertextuality is an organic relationship. In such a relationship, the discourse does not move in just one direction (scar to meaning or meaning to scar) but in multiple directions at the same time. My goal in the remainder of this essay is to suggest that while physical scars inscribe a traumatic event on our bodies, scars are simultaneously writing the body, ensuring that the body's wants, needs, and desires are not ignored. Writing the body, in this context, is a dynamic process that requires the somatic mind in order for the self to be fully integrated.

By acknowledging the place of physical scars in the conversation between mind and body, we can more fully integrate our embodied experiences. In this sense, we can respond to Cixous's plea to "Write! Writing is for you, you are for you; *your body is yours, take it.*"[15] In situating the body as equal to the mind, we are able to re-claim our bodies and re-imagine a history in which women's association with the body is seen as an authentic and valuable experience. My particular scars provide an example of this process: Within the span of six years, I had the two emergency surgeries previously discussed, both in the abdominal region that handles digestion. Both surgeries were caused by inflammation; both concerned either bursting or the possibility of bursting, and both left scars. Additionally, I am facing even more surgery in the same region for similar reasons, and this surgery, of course, would come with a new set of scars. Thinking about my situation with a somatic mind makes it easy to understand the mind-body connection. My psychological and emotional pain has been ingested (swallowed), and my body is refusing to digest it, causing inflammation and agitation along the entire digestive tract. My surgical scars are the nexus of my mind-body connection. In this reading, my mind, my thoughts, and my emotions are crying out to become visible, to be attended to, to be acknowledged, to be cared for in very physical ways. It is possible that even while I am trying to write the body, my body is indeed writing me, forcing attention to be paid to it in its real physical state. My somatic mind is constructing a narrative that is both embodied and psychological/emotional.

The circumstances of my own medical traumas resonate with the imagery Cixous uses when she describes her process of holding things in. She writes: "Time and again, I, too, have felt so full of luminous torrents that I could *burst—burst* with forms much more beautiful than those which are put up in frames and sold for a stinking fortune. And, I, too, said nothing, showed nothing; I didn't open my mouth, I didn't repaint my half of the world. I was ashamed. I was afraid, and I *swallowed* my shame and my fear. I said to myself: *You are mad!*"[16]

Cixous is filled with "luminous torrents" which she describes as "beautiful," yet, she admonishes herself for silencing those torrents, for not speaking up, for not inserting her body, for not claiming her space. In thinking about my abdominal troubles, I cannot help but wonder not only about the negativity I have ingested but also about the powerful voice, my own, that has been muted. What "luminous torrents" have I silenced or have been silenced because of fear of the Medusa? Perhaps my body is making space for something more. What will fill the holes that were left when my organs were removed? Can I fill the void with luminous torrents?

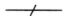

It is not easy to find answers to these questions in traditional scholarship because much of it either ignores the body, women, or both, or equates the female body with disability and disease, not allowing the body much agency.[17] Jay Dolmage, however, has suggested that "rhetoric can reclaim the body,"[18] and he has identified a *metis* rhetoric (named for the Greek goddess, Mêtis) as "cunning, adaptive, *embodied* intelligence"[19] that traditional scholarship has written out of history. To bring *metis* back, we need to re-claim the place of the body in discursive creations of the self. To illustrate how this is possible, Dolmage, like Cixous, turns to Greek mythology.

The goddess, Mêtis, known for her intelligence and cunning, is the first wife of Zeus. While she is pregnant with Zeus's daughter, Athena, Zeus becomes scared that Mêtis's children will be more powerful than him, so he ingests the pregnant Mêtis. Mêtis, however, does not die; Zeus doesn't digest her. Instead she lives inside of Zeus (some say in his belly), and when it is time for Athena to be born, Zeus's head is split open and Athena emerges as a grown adult. For *Mêtis* to have lived in Zeus's belly is a particularly apt metaphor for this essay. If *Mêtis* is Zeus's embodied intelligence, we can imagine that the seat of that intelligence is located in the gut. In this essay, I have been arguing that ignoring my own gut, my own bodily intelligence, has been detrimental to by overall health and well-being. The myth maintains that Mêtis continues to live in Zeus's body, giving him wise counsel. What is interesting about this myth is that Zeus acquires Mêtis's intelligence by physically swallowing her, yet, his body does seem capable of assimilating or digesting her. In this story, Zeus needs to partake of woman—in her full body—to have real strength and intelligence.

—————/—————

Related to the myth of Mêtis the goddess is the idea of metis. According to Dolmage, "[A]s embodied intelligence, *m[e]tis* illuminates a shadowy tangle of body-values, body-denials, and body-power."[20] Debra Hawhee argues that *metis*, as a concept, means that "thought does not just happen within the body, it happens *as* the body."[21] When Zeus swallows Mêtis, he takes her knowledge and cunning into his own body. In this way, body and mind become one. But even though Zeus consumes Mêtis, she retains her self-hood, both by continuing her pregnancy and by remaining an active agent inside of Zeus. Zeus and Mêtis form and intertextual and embodied relationship. Zeus consumes his identity around and through Mêtis's intelligence; Mêtis retains her embodiment by co-creating with Zeus a joint rhetorical body, co-extant with the somatic mind. For Cixous, Mêtis's ability to retain her mind and body while living inside Zeus is that of a heroic woman who has *not* learned to hold her tongue. "For a long time it has been in body that women have responded to persecution, to the familial-conjugal enterprise of domestication, to the repeated attempts at castrating them. Those who have turned their tongues 10,000 times seven times before not speaking are either dead from it or more familiar with their tongues and their mouths than any one else."[22] Mêtis does not keep quiet, and she is not castrated.[23] On the contrary, Mêtis seems to gain power through her tongue and get stronger and more vital when she co-joins with Zeus. Indeed, Mêtis's mind and body empower Zeus: Zeus, a man, is able to give birth, the ultimate embodiment of women's embodied strength. And Mêtis is not silenced. Some say Zeus constantly consulted with her about military and political matters. Zeus and Mêtis even had another child together.

It would be easy for Mêtis to lose herself to Zeus, to hold her tongue; after all, he does EAT her! But the strength of her body and her will (her somatic mind) are so powerful that instead of being absorbed into Zeus, Mêtis and Zeus become integrated. This same kind of integration is necessary to re-embody emotional, psychological, and even physical health today. In narratively constructing and reconstructing the story(ies) of my scars, I have primarily focused on "making sense" in some theoretical way, of the marks on my body. But a *metis*-based interpretation of these scars opens up another way of thinking about these surgeries and their scars.

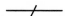

Like Zeus and Cixous, I have swallowed my fear (but not before biting my tongue 10,000 times seven times). Above I have examined one interpretation of these scars: visible markers of inner turmoil, fear and anger and despair made physical. A *metis* based reading provides yet another interpretation. Indeed, to see *metis* as an embodied and wily rhetoric is to give my scars their own voice. Not only do my scars represent the state of my emotional and psychological health but also they are actively communicating that there is something that I need to pay attention to. My scars, in other words, are not mere reactions, inscriptions, or consequences of actions, rather, they are actively constructing meaning; the communication between my body and mind is under constant negotiation. Even as they represent the past, my scars are still refiguring and remapping my future. They are warning me to be aware of what I swallow; I'm not digesting everything I take in and the waste literally needs to go somewhere. As Pennebaker warns: "We are often blind to the psychological causes and correlates to our health problems. Many illnesses and recurring health problems have a psychosomatic component. Awareness or insight into the psychological bases of illness can help in the healing process. If we are aware of the conflicts influencing our bodies, we can act to overcome those conflicts."[24] My scars are my body's way of saying: "you are not paying attention to me. If you won't listen on your own, I will force you to care for me. You are not just a mind; you need me with you on this journey." The consequences of ignoring these types of messages are severe. Our bodies may carry symbols and be symbolic and be socially constructed through discourse, but as many feminists assert, my body (my digestive system, in particular) precedes discourse: it is real and it is angry. I can deconstruct the social construction of my angry colon for the rest of my career, but arguing that "there is no there, there" is not going to make my colon any less angry; future surgery is almost assured and my surgical scars are a constant reminder that my body is corporeal.

My scars are speaking to me about the need to reduce stress and anxiety by making smarter professional and personal choices. While I "knew" in my head that I needed to make these changes before the surgeries, my mind and body were still working as separate entities. The threat of another surgery, this one with more risks and side effects, has shocked my mind into collusion with my body. In this case, my body claimed agency in communicating vital information. If and how we come to enact the somatic mind depends on how well we will be able to stop living in our heads and remember that our brains are covered by skulls which rest upon skeletons that are covered by skin which holds in organs, joints, and muscles which communicate with our brains which make all the things in our bodies work. It is only when we open up these lines of communication to true discursive collaboration that we will begin to fully understand the ability of the body to write itself.

———/———

NOTES

1. In the context of this article, the expression "under my skin" is worth commenting on because the expression encapsulates two ideas central to my argument: things do indeed go on inside the body (under), but also on the surface of the body (skin).
2. See, generally, James Pennebaker.
3. Sarbin, 218.
4. "Angry" and "tortuous" are the exact words doctors have used to describe my colon.
5. "Rhetoric," "discourse," and "discursive practices": In this essay, I use these three terms synonymously as many of the scholars whose work I quote in this essay use these terms interchangeably. However, I do acknowledge that not all scholars would treat these terms as synonyms. A fuller parsing of these terms, however, is beyond the scope of this article.
6. Fleckenstein, 281.
7. Ibid, 284.
8. Dolmage, 3.
9. Ibid.
10. Lunsford, 6.
11. Cixous, 1239.
12. Ibid, 1232-33.
13. Pennebaker, 119.

14. Ibid, 19.
15. Cixous, 1233. Emphasis added.
16. Ibid. Emphasis added.
17. Dolmage, 2-3.
18. Ibid, 5.
19. Ibid.
20. Dolmage, 8.
21. Quoted in Ibid, 6.
22. Cixous 1240.
23. Cixous takes issue with Freud's claim that women have penis envy and the subsequent belief that women are incomplete males because they do not have penises (i.e. women have been castrated).
24. Pennebaker, 24.

BIBLIOGRAPHY

Cixous, Hélène. "The Laugh of the Medusa." (1975). *The Rhetorical Tradition: Readings from Classical Times to the Present*, First Edition. Edited by Patricia Bizzell and Bruce Herzberg. Boston: Bedford Books, 1990. 1232–1244.

Dolmage, Jay. "Metis, Mêtis, Mestiza, Medusa: Rhetorical Bodies across Rhetorical Traditions." *Rhetoric Review 28*, no. 1 (2009): 1–28.

Fleckenstein, Kristie. "Writing Bodies: Somatic Mind in Composition Studies." *College English 61*, no. 3 (1999): 281–306.

Lunsford, Andrea. "On Reclaiming Rhetorica." *Reclaiming Rhetorica: Women in the Rhetorical Tradition*, edited by Andrea Lunsford. Pittsburgh: University of Pittsburgh Press, 1995. 1–8.

Pennebaker, James. *Opening Up: The Healing Power of Expressing Emotions*. New York: Guilford Press, 2012.

Sarbin, Theodore R. "Embodiment and the Narrative Structure of Emotional Life." *Narrative Inquiry 11*, no. 1 (2001): 217–225.

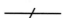

HOLDING ON WHEN I SHOULD'VE LET GO

Emilie Staat

This scar is from a family reunion in Imlay City, Michigan. It was summer 1992 and I was ten years old. I'm not sure who hosted the reunion and I don't think I ever understood how we were related. It didn't particularly matter, then or now, because we went to the reunion for my grandmother's sake—she enjoyed learning about family history and getting together with her siblings and their families, the Michiganders of her blood. There was a pack of kids who were all somehow related to me, mostly boys. Since I was an only child and still considered myself a tomboy, I was pleased to be allowed to run with a familial herd for a few days.

There was a lake on the property, down the hill from the house, with a tall homemade wooden diving board. The ladder leading up to it was steep, with absolutely no incline. It made me think of my favorite movie that had come out the year before, about a girl who is blinded while diving a horse into a large tank of water in Atlantic City. She was stubborn, but also brave, and I wondered if I could be brave enough for this, like her.

I was tall for my age, but ungainly and uncomfortable in my body. I'd gotten my period earlier in the year, a week before my tenth birthday, and I hadn't recovered my creature confidence in my own limbs and flesh. The boy cousins all had it, certainty in their speed and strength and invincibility. I was the youngest, clinging to courage I no longer felt. I had loved to run and swim, but with my new breasts and hips I'd begun to feel a barrier between me and all that I'd once enjoyed. Yet, every part of me felt open, loose, wet. It was like my skin had turned inside out overnight, my internal secrets now constantly presented to the world.

I looked up the ladder as the herd swarmed it ahead of me, some of them leaping twice while I remained uncertainly on the ground. I thought of the girl from the movie, diving with her horse even after she was blinded, and I shakily climbed the ladder. I hauled myself up the rough wood rungs until I cowered on the small platform, high above the large lake below. I wished I had a horse to make the leap with me, to carry me along. I couldn't do it alone.

I turned and scooted down the ladder, which had been built for
ascension only. My bare foot slipped on one of the narrow rungs, damp
from the boy cousins, shedding water like seals as they had flown up it
repeatedly. I flung my arms out to catch myself. It didn't stop my fall, but
my new weight did slow me down. My arms were dragged along the rough
wood, catching splinters and dirt before I collapsed on the sandy grass
below the diving board.

My wrists had become my brakes and were torn up, especially on my
dominant right hand. As my panicked fog retreated, I began to feel the
pain and the fear of how mad the grownups would be. Several of the boys,
queuing up for another jump, circled me.

"Why didn't you just jump off the board?" one of the cousins asked
accusingly as another ran up to the house to get the adults. In his
accusation was the awareness that now we'd probably all get in trouble,
since I was the youngest and a girl. We all knew they were somehow
supposed to be responsible for me and they'd get blamed too for my getting
hurt.

I looked at the swamp of skin and blood on my savaged wrist. I'd heard
some of the girls at school talking about the "right way" to slit your wrists
(*Heathers* had come out four years beforehand and we thrilled with this
forbidden knowledge). I realized that I couldn't have done better if I'd
slashed them on purpose.

Yet I was hurt while actively avoiding pain, holding on for dear life,
when I should have just let go. I couldn't answer my cousin's question,
could barely comprehend it. I realized we didn't speak the same language
anymore, that if being boyish meant you felt no fear or pain, then I was
stuck being a girl forever. I was afraid and I was hurt and I couldn't pretend
I wasn't. I had done it before, prided myself on denying pain when a boy
friend had thrown a baseball at my shin (my leg more bruise than skin for
weeks) and when I'd fallen through the asbestos ceiling of the apartment
complex's laundry room (it had taken quite a lot to get myself up from
the dryers into the ceiling and I was too proud to be hurt). Every tree I'd
climbed had held the potential for pain, but that had never stopped me
before. Pain was a side effect, less than the pride I took in climbing, trying.
But not this time. I wouldn't know how shallow the cuts were until we
cleaned away the blood and dirt and torn flesh. I didn't know I wouldn't die
from this pain. All I knew was there was no pride this time to anesthetize
me: I had climbed, but I hadn't jumped.

The grownups arrived. They were mad, predictably, at the boys. "You know better," they said as they frowned. I thought they were probably, secretly, mad at me for not being brave enough to jump. It was just one of what would become many times I suffered more for holding on, holding back, for not letting go and jumping.

——/——

When I returned to school with the scar, I felt both embarrassed and weirdly proud of this wound that would last, a reminder of a mistake. But though the scar on my right wrist, my writing hand, was ugly for a long time, it eventually faded to a patch of discolored skin that only I knew was there. It became far too easy to forget how I had been marked as I'd transitioned from confident creature to uncertain woman. I never remembered until it was too late and kept making the same mistake, in different forms. As an adult, I got a tattoo over the scar, not to hide it, but to transform it into something that would always remind me to embrace my openness and my wounds. To let go. To leap.

——/——

Socks

Heidi Kim

I have never really known what to make of my scar. I've never thought of it
as affecting my life, but then again, I can't remember a day without it, or a
time when my mother could pat my leg without mourning over it. It's just
there, and it's not that bad, since I don't care very much about appearance;
or do I not care about appearance because I've always had such a terrible
scar?

My scar covers the lower two-thirds of the back of my left calf, in a
slightly darker, blotchy oval, uneven and shiny. I was born with a large dark
splotch there, like a giant mole, and the doctors convinced my mother that
it was probably precancerous. She wanted to take me to New York to have
it done at one of the big hospitals, but they talked her out of that as well.
So they did the skin graft when I was a few months old, and made a pretty
bad job of it, as far as I can tell. Recently, however, I found out that maybe
it has been impacting me all along more than I ever thought; a physical
therapist told me that the operation had shaved off a bit of muscle and
had probably thrown the whole leg slightly off all my life. This explains the
misaligned tendon in my knee that sometimes makes a delightful snap,[1]
and the disconcerting hitch-click in my hip when I do *pavanamuktasana*
pose on the left side. Because of it, I will almost certainly never be able to
run a marathon, but then again, I doubt that I ever would have, anyway.
Nonetheless, this bit of information has made me think recently about
whether or not my scar has shaped my life in ways I hadn't recognized.

There have been very few other obvious effects; it used to ache terribly
in hot baths, so I avoided whirlpools for several years, but more recently, as
the scar seems to have settled down a bit more, I have discovered that as it
turns out, I don't particularly like hot baths, so I'm not really missing out
on something that might be upsetting to someone else.

I remember absolutely nothing about my scar or the social experience of
it until about second grade. My mother resolutely dressed me in knee-high
socks if I was in shorts or skirts, because she felt so terrible about it that she
wanted it covered all the time (a good example, parents or parents-to-be, of

---

1. When I first mentioned it, around age twelve, my mother had me do the snap
   for my pediatrician at my next checkup (just a squat will do it). He looked
   thrilled and said, "Do it again!" It's quite a snap.

inflicting your own anxieties on your children, and no, I don't blame her, because she really felt *that terrible* about it.

When I was younger, she used to pet the scar and say that she must have done something bad in a past life and was being punished). The knee-high socks were white, thin, very elastic, often with little lacey translucent patterns woven into them. I don't suppose they were cheap, and they possibly represented somewhat of a financial splash for my parents at that time. Nonetheless, considering that my favorite item of apparel at that age was a yellow sweatshirt with a sparkly lion's head printed on it, I did not look like the height of 80s style. I might as well have gone to school carrying a shovel for the mean girls to beat me to death with before they dug my grave.

There was one classmate in particular—Amy was her name— who tormented me constantly. I don't even remember how, I just remember that it was constant and loud. Just to shut her up, I finally wore my mother down and got different socks. My mother was only persuaded when I told her that I had been rolling the socks down once I got to school, anyway. I had made an art form out of it; I used to roll them very slowly and precisely to create little white donuts around my ankles. With the blessed perversity of childhood, nobody made any fun of me for that. By then, it was the late 80s, and big slouch socks were in, so my mother was happy that "The Scar" was at least a little covered up. Better yet, *double* slouch socks came in, the oversock in a contrasting color slouched a few inches lower than the undersock. My color combination of choice was black and fluorescent pink, matched by *double* scrunchies.[2]

After second grade, there's a black hole of sorts in my scar memory. In the tweens and teens, people would ask about it when we hit shorts season, but that was usually it; sometimes, someone would kindly try to tell me I had dirt on my leg and then get terribly embarrassed. (This still happens, though very rarely.) The older I got, the longer it generally took people to get around to asking; sometimes I would volunteer the information if I could feel them looking at it. (This polite looking also still happens, but even more rarely. Perhaps as we get older, so many of us have scars that they're not so noteworthy anymore.)

There is a piece of collateral damage, though, that those of you who have had skin grafts or know about them will have noticed that I have thus far omitted in this tale. The skin has to come from somewhere. Where do you take skin off a two-month-old baby? Apparently, from the lower

---

2. I'm from New Jersey, by the way.

right ass cheek.[3] Remarkably, considering how much I swam as a child, I don't remember any comments about my butt. I think 80s cuts on little girls' bathing suits might have been modest enough that almost none of it showed. Regardless, I never thought about the second scar much and don't think I even knew what it looked like until I was twenty-one. I realize that this might sound unbelievable, but nobody was doing yoga back then, so twisting around to look at it was out of the question, and I'd never bothered to stand naked with my back to a mirror.

The first real opinion I got on my ass scar came from a close college friend who had always been very openly sad about my calf scar. It was either in the dressing room at a Banana Republic or on the beach in Barcelona on our post-college backpacking trip, I can't remember which. She took a look at my ass and told me that the scar looked a bit like cellulite. She then refused to speak to me for a couple of days because she was so resentful that I didn't have any actual cellulite and, even worse, didn't know what cellulite was.[4] Odd trade-off: lumpy scar, no cottage cheese fat.

You may have already foreseen still more collateral damage, or a dilemma, at any rate. What's it like for a partner, revealing that lumpy cellulite-looking scar on the ass? I was having a conversation once with another female friend about disclosure to intimate partners—not STDs, but physical disclosures, like circumcision (or lack thereof) for men, which was what she had recently discovered about the man she was dating. I said that I always warned men about my ass, even if they were just going to see me in a bikini. "I don't want them to be *surprised*," I said. Or worse yet, to wonder and politely not ask. She found this very strange, but I have always found that honesty is indeed the best policy.[5] The only danger in it is that a man will tend to imagine that it's worse than it actually is, so the warning has to come about an instant before the reveal, so that he can't freak himself out. However, it is very entertaining to watch him bravely bracing himself to be noble and high-minded.

---

3. Come to think of it, this must mean it was at Banana Republic, because I don't think we could have survived Barcelona without speaking to each other. The hostel we stayed in was full of whores and pickpockets. It sounds like a Dickens novel, but I'm serious. Prostitutes lived there.

4. You have to say 'ass' in this situation. 'Buttock' sounds like Chaucer; 'ass' has the twang of humor or defiance, especially if you have central Jersey vowels.

5. I'd made a policy of disclosing the scar, weirdly enough, after learning that another friend—no longer a friend, not entirely incidentally—didn't disclose to men she slept with that she had HPV. It turned me overly scrupulous.

My scar still hurts me almost every day, but I don't mean emotionally. There is still a vague voice in my head that has to speak up after I shower: "Moisturize before it gets tight," or "Scar's itching, Lubriderm." In the summer, it just pulls a bit; in the winter, at its worst, it can be a constant, stabbing pain. I keep a bottle of lotion in my desk drawer at work.

It's an inconvenience that I live with, like people whose nails break or lips chap or hearts burn. In spite of the occasional pain, I have never cared enough to see a plastic surgeon about it. I have never cared enough about the one on my ass even to call it a scar—I only refer to one scar, singular. It does make me roam the lotion aisle at Target with a constantly acquisitive eye.

Ultimately, though, there is the desire to find some way that the scar has shaped or changed me, however slight it may be. It may well have taught me how to handle awkward social situations, romantic relationships, or peer pressure (switching socks was about the last time I caved to it). Even though I can't remember much about the scar itself from my childhood, I do know that I had to explain it all the time as soon as I was old enough to be asked. And it is, as you may have thought to yourself at the beginning of this piece, a very dull story. Savvy people recognize that it's a skin graft, and they always asked me if it was from a burn. I used to wish it were a burn. I used to imagine how I would have gotten said burn. A car accident, that was my favorite one;[6] I tried to imagine knocking something off the stove, but I ran into the plausibility problem of how I would get burned down the lower half of the back of my calf and nowhere else. I thought maybe my mom could knock something off the stove and splash me, but that seemed a bit mean, even in imagination, when she already felt so bad about the scar. I invented worlds that ended with the destruction of my lower left leg; I inherited kingdoms when I was recognized because of my scar as the long-lost kidnapped/shipwrecked/forgotten princess.[7] I wished for it to have a *story*. So, I suppose, the common ground for many of us with large visible scars is that scars give us practice at telling stories, whether to ourselves or to others, and that is something that stays with you even as you outgrow the burdens of childhood, knee-high socks, and mean girls.

---

6. I had, excitingly, been in a car accident at the age of five that totaled our Volkswagen Rabbit but left us all unharmed. As I had a very undramatic childhood, it was probably the only disaster that I knew how to imagine.

7. I stole this idea from Joan Aiken's *Black Hearts in Battersea*, which I didn't particularly enjoy, but it features some long-lost nobility recognized by the white tuft of hair amid their black curls.

(Un)holy Hands

Jason Wiest

Carol Frerichs shrieked like she'd just seen Satan, but there really wasn't much I could piously do to blunt her alarm.

We were standing at the altar of the First United Methodist Church in Lodgepole, Nebraska, a village of few more than 300 people. The day's service had ended, and Carol's daughter and I stood in a receiving line with the rest of the teenagers who'd just been confirmed as members of the church. If the past several months of Wednesday night "youth group" meetings were actually a test of our obedience to the cross and not just an activity to keep us out of trouble, the next moment was surely God giving me the pop quiz of my life.

"What's on the back of your hand?" Carol asked.

Morning sunlight beamed on me from the gigantic stained glass window like I was getting the holy trinity's third degree. I knew that telling the truth, especially to someone like Carol—a motorcycle-riding, say-what-you-feel, do-what-you-want type who was rarely seen in church and not a Lodgepole native—would potentially present me with the biggest dermatological embarrassment of my entire acne-prone life. But we were standing at an altar. There, choosing a response felt like a major afterlife decision, and if everything I'd been learning in confirmation classes were true, I couldn't risk telling a lie—especially the lie I'd mastered.

How many times before, when asked about my hand, had I feigned a shameful look before breaking eye contact with my inquisitor and settling in to the solemnity the situation never failed to create? After casting that dark mood, I'd lightly touch the three or four mostly circular scars on the back of my hand, drawing a mask of sorrow over my face. Without saying a word, I'd taken control of the conversation. It was a prodigal display of the art of body language, even if the canvas was badly scarred.

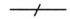

"I don't know. I guess when I misbehaved when I was little, my mom would burn me with a cigarette." With a slight jolt into a more rigid posture, I'd hurry my eyes back to direct contact with my inquisitor's, saying, "But she's not like that anymore or anything."

Pity often looked back at me, sometimes even the watery-eyed with whispered coos of solidarity kind. And there were probably a few people who looked back at me in horror over my mom's alleged actions, too. As bad as it sounds, those moments of emotional puppeteering were satisfying self-defense. After the tale, I had each nosy scar interrogator right where I wanted them. With this backdrop, when I revealed the truth, they would be off-kilter enough that their instinctive reaction of disgust could be disguised with a layer of laughter or confusion, or horror at the mother of my imagination.

But Carol never got the chance to mask her reaction, because I did not present her with my tried-and-true, carefully scripted drama. For me on that day, standing in a beam of colored light from above, deciding not to call my dear mother a despicable monster was a WWJD no-brainer.

"They're from warts," I said, unleashing Carol's audible terror on the sanctuary.

The Lord was the shepherd I hadn't wanted that Sunday. He had madeth me lie down in wart-infested pastures and then ledeth judgmental parishioners past me. Carol's commotion caused those waiting to shake the hand in question to wonder what was wrong, and I spent a good piece of the morning telling the truth in different ways, searching for the version that would mitigate the emotional scarring taking place within my vulnerable adolescent soul.

There seemed to be no way to be honest and charming at the same time. These scars didn't come with an action-adventure story as did the inoffensive bike crash scar on my knee, a body part unintrusive to others. When people asked follow-up questions beyond the origin of that scar, they even got a bonus comedic twist: my dad had applied butter to the wound, while we both tried not to faint at the sight of my blood.

Because these scars were from warts, it seemed I could either be honest, or I could be presentable. Somehow, even the scar on my face is palatable to people, now that it isn't a cystic pimple. Back then, it attracted enough ridicule to make it the biggest crisis of my year in 7th grade, but as a scar, it goes mostly unnoticed, with the rare inquiry resulting in the type of favorable review usually reserved for beauty marks. (Which, I might remind, are just moles on your face.) Beauty's where you find it, as they say. Take it from someone who knows them like the back of their hand: back-handed wart scars are not where many people find beauty.

Instead, people found fear in them, and I, rejection. Before they were eaten away with physician-applied acid in a multi- day-long, hurt-so-good process, the warts had briefly situated me as a pariah at school. They marked me as the carrier of a potential contagion, or at least an easy target for teenage ridicule. Maybe my skin was just too thin at that age. Either way, the truth had been used against me to make me feel as though I were repulsive.

To be fair, there were a few rare instances of compassion and acceptance. Some church folk shook my now extra sweaty, wart-scarry hand anyway without asking questions or making remarks. By then, though, either God-given ESP or my own paranoia had rendered me their secret abhorrence. Trapped, I endured far more judgment that I anticipated that day. After all, this was my confirmation, not my funeral.

Years after the day I joined the church, I began to wonder if an outsider like Carol among a homogenous population like the Lodgepole First United Methodist Church congregation might only have been acting horrified, either for her own amusement or some other purpose. Whether she intended to or not, by thrusting my scars into the spotlight, she taught me a real-world lesson in a faith-based place.

Some people considered the truth—my truth—to be an abomination. But the reality is that scars aren't contagious, nor anything over which we have much control. At the time, though, that knowledge was overshadowed by my obsession with what other people thought. There I was, desperately trying to contrive other people's reactions to spare myself from shame and embarrassment, when all I had to do was stand firm in the truth and know that there was no reason to be ashamed or embarrassed. When I stopped trying to mold what other people thought of me, I could observe how they interacted with me, and then make my own decisions. It was like Carol had gotten off her motorcycle and showed me how to stop riding bitch.

However, I didn't learn that lesson the day Carol taught it to me. I'm certain I watched contemptuously that Sunday as she retreated down the aisle, likely headed for her royal blue house on dusty Bates Boulevard and into its dark recesses of flea market Victorian décor. It was a blighted home that stuck out in our monotonous town as much as she did —a scar upon our little village. Perhaps she was so rarely seen in church because she was enlightened enough to seek acceptance from herself instead of others. I fold my scarred hands and pray.

———/———

THE LAST MARK OF BOYHOOD

Maurice Carlos Ruffin

I was seven when it occurred to me I wasn't immortal. The lucky among us recall a time before our first serious injury, before the cut that hurts forever and introduces us to the general state of affairs.

A child of the 80s, I was brought up in a walled subdivision called Kingswood on the edge of Bayou Sauvage National Wildlife Preserve in New Orleans. More than anything, I associate Kingswood with wholesome hijinks, the archetypal American childhood depicted on *The Andy Griffith Show*, *Lassie*, and *Dennis the Menace*.

Kingswood was a new development, so new that the northern half was still under construction when we moved in. Most of the buyers were young, working-class families with small children. This meant I had dozens of possible playmates. But my best buds around then were two guys whose houses were practically back-to-back. I'll call the guys Duke and Oliver. Oliver's mama was a strict disciplinarian who unfairly forced us to wash goop, grease, and grime from our hands before eating the donuts that were ever-present at their kitchen table. Duke's mama was a born-again Christian given to pulling the three of us down to our knees for impromptu prayer sessions. And when we sometimes scuffled in my den, my mama, observing us through the kitchen serving window, would raise an eyebrow and say, "Be good." None of the mamas stopped us from coming up with get-rich-quick schemes like selling our coloring book pages to grown folk at a dollar a pop.

One late spring day, the three of us gathered with a pile of rusty nails, cracked hammers, and warped, wooden planks. We were going to make scooters, not for profit, but for our own amusement. The design was so simple that even small children could build them. And so we did.

Two wooden planks for the floor and mast. One smaller board for the handlebars. A pair of roller skates for locomotion. We wanted to get a little assembly line going, to make a dozen of them, but we were so excited by completing the first one that we never got around to making any more. Still, we did a good job with the one we built. The thing actually worked! Duke zoomed down his driveway and into traffic. Then Oliver did the same. I begged for my turn. No mamas in sight.

Can I tell you that waiting at the top of Duke's driveway, perched on my brand new, nuclear-powered scooter was one of the defining moments of my young life? This was just the beginning of my long-dreamed-of career as an astronaut. Soon, I'd voyage to Pluto as the captain of my own spaceship.

I steadied myself and pushed off. Wind coursed across my body, my buddies were left earthbound back on the driveway, and I imagined myself streaking into outer space like The Shuttle.

But I didn't achieve orbit that day. Somewhere near the street, I hit a hidden crease in the sidewalk. I was heavier than my friends, and my weight didn't allow me to glide over the imperfections in the concrete left behind by the construction crew, who were probably watching the fiasco from atop a crane boom halfway across town, laughing.

My fall wasn't spectacular. I didn't topple head over heels or go flying into the adjacent yard. I simply fell forward *splat!* on my hands and knees. I was used to falling and skinning the flesh from whatever part of my body grated the ground. Small wounds and scars are the currency of boyhood. If you don't get hurt often, you're probably not having much fun.

I was more worried about the scooter. Did I break it? We'd spent, like, two hours on it, which was practically a week in kid time. But the scooter was fine. In fact, checking my face and hands, I was fine, too—or so I thought.

No one asked if I was alright. Maybe they were in shock. They just stared at my leg. I had a gash, opened like a small mouth, just above my right knee. And too, there was an impressive amount of blood was gushing from it. I wondered how this happened. Then I saw the culprit. A long nail jutted from the mast board like a horn. This sort of thing never happened to astronauts.

Having put together cause and effect, and seeing that I now had what appeared to be an asteroid-sized hole in my leg, I did what any red-blooded boy would have done. I cried like a baby. Great galloping sobs. I couldn't see or hear for some time. Plus, it hurt!

Eventually, I found myself in Duke's back yard with him and Oliver watching me in pity, shaking their heads, possibly wondering if they could have my action figures if I died. Some other kids had come over to see what the hoopla was and scampered away when they realized what the hoopla was.

Duke's dad appeared in the doorway. He was a policeman and about eleven feet tall. He also had a huge Jheri Curl, so that overall he looked like a massive talking tree.

"What's all this crying?" he asked, kneeling in front of me. He took a gander at the problem. Surely, in all his years on the force he'd never seen anything so gruesome as my leg wound.

"Stop," he said. Stop? What did he mean *stop*? I was mortally wounded. A goner. My days numbered. I'd never thought about death much before that day, and realized the consequences of my impending demise: my poor, sainted mother would have to make do with my dumb, older brother. I really wanted to tell Duke's dad that I couldn't stop crying. But I couldn't stop crying.

"You ain't dying." He pinched my shoulder. "Be a man."

I imagine that men have said this to boys since prehistoric times, since little Grod had a finger bitten off by a wolf. Maybe the phrase is a sort of incantation that, when spoken with the proper amount of testosterone-fueled conviction, transforms the hearer from a tender child to a young adult instantaneously.

I stopped crying.

To my surprise, I didn't die. And eventually, the gash in my leg healed. It left a lozenge-shaped blemish, about the size of a large vitamin, which is visible even now.

But I often recall those days and my irreversible transformation. I remember the women who raised us and did their best to protect us from the dangers of the world and from ourselves. And I remember the men who taught us what the world expected of us.

———/———

THE PRY BAR

Philip Martin

"It was cathartic," you say now
when you tell our demolition story to guests
who wonder at the openness
of our rooms and how they got that way.
We took a sledge, smashed the iron tub
to shards, ripped down walls and
in the evenings sat on plastic tarp
and wept for other lives foreclosed.
And though I did not know myself
I would tell you (I would promise you)
we were all right and would be still
after writing the carpenter's check
and paying for the cabinets
custom-ordered for our kitchen.
"Numbers are just numbers," I decreed,
in my best basso big boy voice.

Then one day I stuck our ripping tool
—the pry bar—in the bathroom wall.
It caught; I strained and pulled it out
reaping a whirlwind of drywall smut.
When the cloud cleared, the pry bar was
stuck deep in my side, beneath my ribs.
"Forthwith there came out blood and water,"
I remember thinking to myself.

You cleaned the gash with peroxide.
It never stung. We bandaged it
and when it healed it left on my skin
a raised filament, a white seam.
That, months later, was remarked upon
by Doctor Stephen Tilley
who asked me how this tidy scar came to be.
I shared the tale. He doubted me:
It didn't happen like that, he said:
It must have been in Mexico
when you stepped in with common sense

to referee a dispute between
two criminal biker chieftains.
They shook hands in the cantina,
your work was done, but on the sidewalk
a prospect looking to make his bones
shivved you between the ribs.

Your forgiveness didn't save him.
They buried his parts in the alkaline
wasteland of del Notre de Sonoran and
when they dropped you across the border
at the American hospital, they warned you:
 "Never speak of this, mi amigo,
tell them you did it remodeling."

And so I tell the pry bar story.

Now, on the occasions I touch the scar
and am forced back unwittingly,
it is Tilley's version that prevails
over the dull dumb domestic facts
of the demolition accident.
I believe it —
for there were times when I was younger,
more afraid, and full of hunger.

Before you, there was the Christmas in Chicago
when the kid with the screwdriver
and the broken teeth and broken pride
tried to take my money
outside of married student housing
at the U. of C.: It was his blood,
not mine, on the sidewalk,
embeamed by police flashlights,
leading South down Cottage Grove.
I had hurt him.
And she—the one before you—was frightened
by my fury and desperation
by my unregulated eyes.
By the way I kept on hitting him
after I caught him in the doorway.
I went to a hotel that night
and rolled over in my mind,
hard and unproveable theories about myself.

She and I were having our troubles then.
It might have been I wanted to die
defending her; just to show
I wasn't like the others that
she sometimes spoke to me about
the wormboys and the brutish men
 like the one who held the pistol
(unloaded, she believed and hoped)
to his own head as she fellated him.

What was it *she* had wanted?
Something unvoiceable and cruel?
Did she want to cry for me struck down
and bleeding, my life stuff leaching out,
her poor martyred blondboy husband
killed and gone away forever?
It was my fault, my striving,
my persistent male unsated need.
I could have given him the money.
Numbers are just numbers, after all.

And our scars are just evidence of old hurts,
impotent as bills long paid
languishing in old file boxes,
good for nothing but reminding us
of times we thought we had it rough.
Sometimes beneath my shirt I find it,
the spot where the pry bar caught me.
I rub it for luck; now I know:
It was just a scratch.
I see now I lived for you.
Somehow I found the leverage
to make the discontentment give,
to snap it into dust and powder.
I am glad for the murder
of the man I might have been.
The explosion
that hurtled me into your arms.
That put the pry bar in my hand.

———/———

MY SCHMISS

James S. Baumlin

"Identification is known to psychoanalysis as the earliest expression
of an emotional tie with another person" [Freud, "Group Psychology,"
Standard Edition 18:105]. It plays a part in the early history of the
Oedipus complex, and Freud describes how the young boy reacts as
regards his father: 'he would like to grow like him and be like him,
and take his place everywhere. We may say simply that he takes his
father as his ideal' [*Standard Edition* 18:105]. . . . [The boy] then has
to deal with what psychoanalysis calls the normal Oedipal situation,
in which his masculine identification takes on a hostile colouring
with respect to his father-as-rival. . . . This means of course that his
identification is ambivalent in nature.

—Jean-Michel Quinodoz, *Reading Freud* (198)

———/———

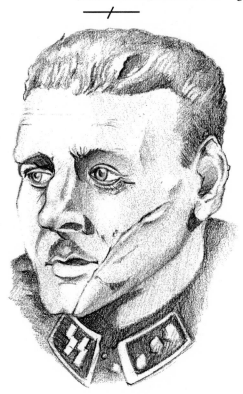

The Schmiss (or *Mensurschmiß*, "dueling scar") in the accompanying
sketch belonged to Otto Skorzeny (1908–1975), an SS colonel and expert
in espionage. However lionized in photographs, his Schmiss is not my
Schmiss—that is, the one that I imagined for myself in middle school,
around the age of thirteen. His Schmiss, while impressive, isn't particularly
clean: some muscular contortion and a semicircular sweep of his
opponent's dueling sword (or *Mensurschläger*—it was Skorzeny's tenth duel,

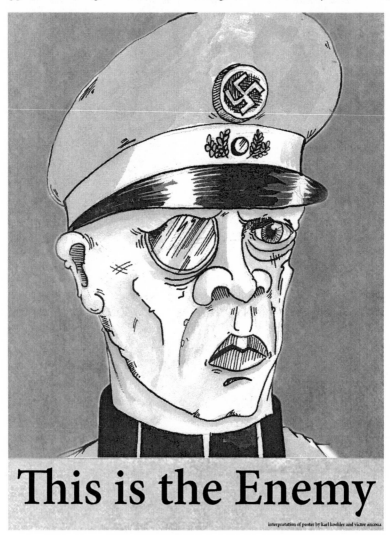

This is the Enemy

interpretation of poster by karl koehler and victor ancona

by the way) made for a broken and uneven cut. *Mine* would have been
a clean razor-like cut starting at the mouth's left edge and following the
jawline, curling upward just before the ear. Colonel Skorzeny's portrait is
also lacking an ornament of cultural importance: surely no self-respecting
SS officer would have been called well-dressed without a monocle in his
right eye—the perfect complement to the Schmiss on his left cheek.

I teach college-level courses in memoir-writing nowadays, in which
coming-of-age stories are a common theme. And I have asked students if
they know what a Schmiss is.

"A what?" they say.

"Oh, the Schmiss survives in popular culture," I tell them. There's
Doctor Evil from the Austin Powers movies, who is himself a parody of
Ernst Stavro Blofeld, head of SPECTRE and James Bond's archenemy in
Thunderball (1965), among other Ian Fleming films. (Strictly speaking,
their Schmisses are on the wrong cheek and aim the wrong direction,
vertically rather than horizontally.) As to the monocle, there's Colonel
Klink of *Hogan's Heroes*, a television comedy that began its six-year run
in 1965. (Again, strictly speaking, the colonel wears his monocle on the
wrong eye.) What surprises me still is that, as an adolescent coming of
age in the 1960s on the East Coast of the United States of America—
specifically, in Perth Amboy, New Jersey—I found myself searching
for images of rugged masculinity and somehow found them in the
quintessentially German monocle and facial scar.

I've assumed that my father was German in ancestry, though I know
next to nothing about his family: he didn't speak much, and he died when
I was in my twenties. So I pretty much invented a history for him and, in
part, for myself. I'm pretty sure that my father, who served in World War II,
had himself been taught to scorn the monocle-sporting, scarred image that
so fascinated me in adolescence. I remember watching the televised trial
of Adolf Eichmann on an old black-and-white TV set in my grandfather's
bedroom. I was in first grade: I can confirm the year, as a web-search tells
me that the trial took place in 1961. I can't confirm the next anecdote,
but my mother tells me that, when I was introduced to my second-grade
teacher, my first words were, "Don't tell anyone, but my father's a Nazi."
(I assume they laughed at that, and I assume that I puzzled over their
laughter.) I guess that, at a young age, I had identified Germanness with the
images of Nazism that still circulated freely throughout popular culture, in
films and on television.

I am too, too aware of the Freudian implications of all this. There's guilt and a vaguely Oedipal identification invested in this childhood fantasy that sees one's father as a Nazi, watches televised trials of Nazi war criminals, and yet imagines oneself with a monocle and Schmiss.

A further complication in my adolescent self-image comes from my mother's side, which is Polish. We were, as an extended family, far more Polish than German, given that my mother's parents were Polish immigrants and Polish was spoken in their home. And we attended a Polish-Catholic church. This was before the reforms of Vatican II (1962–1965), so the liturgy was conducted in Latin and Greek while the sermon was in Polish: as a result, I spent church-time mostly daydreaming. (My mother never taught her children Polish. Possibly she wanted us to be American exclusively, but she also used the language against us, as a means of excluding her children from adult conversations. I wish now that she had taught us; in contrast, I went on to study German at the graduate level.) When not daydreaming, I sat admiring the church architecture—though without understanding. Built in the height of the Depression, its granite and sandstone magnificence bespeaks the pious sacrifice of immigrants. The stained glass—imported from Europe—told the history of Poland through the Middles Ages to the Napoleonic Wars. I didn't know this as an adolescent; I didn't know the names of the saints and soldiers and kings depicted. I didn't know that the history of Poland after Napoleon was one of partition and conquest. I *did* know that the Polish horse cavalry folded to German Panzers in a mere two weeks of Blitz Krieg (television documentaries taught me this) and that the Russians ultimately replaced the Germans as occupiers (this the Cold-War television news taught me).

At any rate, I seem to have thought simplistically of Poles as a conquered people and of Germans as good at conquering, though habitually overreaching in their ambitions. I haven't lived in New Jersey since finishing college, and it wasn't until my early fifties that I understood things better. Attending a funeral back in Perth Amboy, I looked at the stained glass with fresher eyes. The message was clear: Don't forget. And I thought back to a yearly parade, when I played the trombone (badly) in the Perth Amboy High School Marching Band. We marched behind a half-dozen Polish freedom fighters who had immigrated after the war, each dressed in a uniform of some sort and carrying a heavy old rifle. We'd march up to a stone monument, play the Polish national anthem (very badly), and a single trumpeter would play taps. The Polish freedom fighters would then fire off a ragged salute. In my senior year, I noted that there were fewer freedom fighters marching with us, but the elegiac cause for that never came to mind.

Jeszcze Polska nie zginęła—"Poland has not yet perished"—vs.
Deutschland über alles: I have, just over the past few years, learned
something of the history of the Polish freedom fighters. I have learned
that there's something nobler in resisting conquest than in conquering. I
probably knew this all along, but the adolescent version of myself didn't
know how to articulate it.

"Now what," the reader might ask, "does this seeming internal warfare
between my Polish and my German blood have to do with an essay on
scars—or, more specifically, on a 'duelling scar' *that I do not have?*" I hope
the following serves to explain.

———✝———

The real power of *Oedipus Rex* lies not in the fact that it illustrates
the Oedipus complex—that Oedipus was oedipal—but that it depicts
a troubling and seemingly universal dimension of human behavior;
the way we unwittingly create the fate we fear and abhor. Oedipus,
like most of us, falls victim to what he frantically strove to avoid. We
identify with Oedipus not because we wish to possess one parent and
eliminate the other, but because we too end up precisely where we
didn't want to...

—Jeffrey B. Rubin, "The Real Oedipal Complex"

Close to a dozen years ago, I was seeing a sports-massage therapist for a
frozen shoulder. As the therapist rolled his forearm back and forth over the
tendon to release "trigger points" that had gotten stuck, he asked, "Where'd
you get that scar?" Two inches long and folded inward like pursed lips,
it sits near the top of my right deltoid where the therapist was working.
Several years prior, I had had a lipoma removed: just a lipoma, a benign
fatty lump.

"Oh, an old war wound," I said lazily, not interested in small-talk.

"Shrapnel?" he rejoined, his interest piqued.

Now I knew I had made a mistake—and a big mistake at that, since the
Missouri Ozarks (where I live and teach) seems to send more than its share
of young men and women into the military and I suspect that my therapist
(a big man in his early fifties who knew his job well and had worked on
some heavy-weight clients, including defensive linemen of the Kansas City
Chiefs) had seen his share of scars. Whether he had been in the military
himself, I don't know (again, like my father, I'm not into small-talk); but
I knew immediately to atone for my evasive non-answer and to declare
admiration (genuine) for those who have fought in fact and have shed
blood in the fighting. Mine, simply, was a thoughtless response. And the

therapist didn't seem to hold it against me. But I don't have to be told that one never lies about things military, scars especially.

And I found myself wondering: why did I answer in that way, however lazily and unthinking? And I found an answer of sorts that lay in an old set of narratives—some told to me, some told by me—all proceeding from an adolescent premise: that one's sense of selfhood (for which, in my case, read early manhood) is to be valued against the "going rate" of one's physical scars. And, habitually, I have told lies about my own.

Since age thirteen, I've never not worked—though some might wonder if being an English professor counts in the same way as delivering soda, which my father did for much of his adulthood. Taking pride in things blue-collar, I remind my students (many of whom are first-generation college students, coming from working-class backgrounds) that it's hard work, not brilliance, that will get them through. And some of the stories that I tell, particularly in classes on memoir-writing, are about working in a soda plant with my father—a work place that was really too dangerous for the scrawny thirteen-year-old that I was.

I got hurt more than a few times there, though only one accident left its physical mark—as a result, the fingernails on my left hand are unnaturally large and domed. I had been sitting on an aluminum birch beer barrel with arms dangling at my sides, and a full barrel—which some fool had dropped or let loose—came rolling down a ramp, smashing my left hand against my barrel-seat. I remember blood spurting from the tips of my fingers (which I didn't know was possible: at times like these, we experience our bodies at a distance—until pain reminds us that we're their inhabitants still). And I remember my father walking me over to the plant's industrial-sized sink to wash off my hand. As we walked, he plucked the fingernails off one by one, as they had popped off and were hanging, each by some broken skin. I've mentioned pain but I don't have any recollection of it; my only memories are audial (hearing the rolling barrel smashing against my barrel seat with my hand in between) and visual (seeing what fingers look like without nails). When I tell this story, it's to remind my students where I come from, work-wise. In the blue-collar world of my father, a man's labor is supposed to leave its marks.

The soda plant is the only true story that I tell about scars; then again, I have only one other scar that's not usually hidden by clothing. And it's not much of a scar. It's a slender ridge about three-quarters of an inch long down the knuckle of my right middle finger. The scar stands out when I make a fist, though I would likely have to point it out for people to see it. I got it playing on the schoolyard in seventh grade: the urban public schoolyards in Perth Amboy were entirely asphalt, cheap to maintain but rough on one's knuckles and knees and elbows. And I have, indeed, lied about it in several variations over the years.

"See that scar, there?" I'd say up close to a student: "That's where the Polish nun whacked me on the knucks with a ruler." Nowadays, catechism classes—and nuns with rulers—seem to fascinate my mostly WASPish students. Throughout my middle-school years I spent Friday afternoons being chauffeured to the local Polish-Catholic school for confirmation lessons. Not all Polish nuns wielded rulers back then, but some did, and they seemed determined to beat religion into the heathen public-schoolers who showed up once weekly. At the least, they nipped daydreaming in the bud. I don't remember much of the catechism—

Why did God make us?

God made us to show his goodness and to make us happy with Him in heaven . . .

—but I do remember being whacked for looking out the window, daydreaming. It was a beautiful spring afternoon and I had already put in a full day in public school. To spend yet another hour in any classroom for any reason seemed cruel and unusual. The nun certainly didn't draw blood, but that doesn't mean that I made it unscathed though the religious teachings of my childhood.

I have made other stories out of that scarred knuckle, like the time I "creamed a gypsy" while sightseeing in Rome. I was in my early thirties. I did, in fact, *push* a gypsy—a young man, tall, dark-featured—who was reaching into a traveling companion's pocket for a wallet. I had noticed the gypsy shadowing my tourist group and began shadowing him in turn, so that the moment he made his move, I made mine. But I pushed him, I didn't punch him. The fact is that I've never tried to punch anyone since middle school, and even back then I couldn't find it in myself to hurt anyone deliberately. Shoving and wrestling are defensive maneuvers, and I've done my share of shoving. But knuckle-punching?

Once while in seventh grade, I took a challenge to fight someone after school. It was me with my twin brother and him with some dueling "second" of his own. I think he was Puerto Rican, though all my friends back then were either Jewish or Puerto Rican so race wasn't an issue. I don't remember the cause of our *duellum*, though I assume it involved some insult. He threw the first punch, hitting me in the eye hard enough to cause a shiner (which, the next day, I did my best to hide with my mother's makeup). At this point, my brother stepped behind and put him in a full nelson, pinning his arms behind his back. (We used to watch pro wrestling on TV and I still remember the names of the wrestling moves.) I could have pummeled him, I guess. But I told my brother to let him go and we left.

At home, I had to make up a story about how I had held my own. My brother didn't feel like contradicting me, and my father nodded approvingly as he ate supper. As a young boy, one remembers the stories told by or about one's father, like the time at the local bowling alley when my father broke a man's arm for flirting with my mother. Anger management was achieved with one's fist: so I was taught, as were my friends.

"Yeah, our pop was so angry at us that he put his fist through the wall at the supermarket." So a friend told me, in almost hushed awe, not remorseful for whatever he had done to anger his father but simply over the latter's show of force. An awesome fatherly force it appeared, both to him and to me. I remember his father being a big hulky man who drank often and a lot, and I suspect (looking back) that alcohol added to the force of his punch.

Now flash-forward from the supermarket to an apartment in Fort Worth: I was in my late twenties and with my soon-to-be wife. An older colleague from where I was teaching at the time had come over for supper and, a bit heavily into his cups, had made an offensive declaration (for which he would apologize the next day). I parried his insult: his answer, I believe, was "*Touché.*" I didn't fly into an immediate rage (as I had been taught); I didn't offer to punch my colleague or break his arm. Still, the image of a friend's drunken father breaking sheetrock flashed through my mind and I resolved to reassert my manhood by punching a wall in the apartment hallway.

This turned out to be a life-lesson. I now know that, in order to break through a sheetrock wall effectively, you have to be very drunk, fairly strong, moderately to severely stupid, and considerably *lucky* (so as to hit the wall *between the studs*). I seem to have fallen short in all categories, since I broke neither the wall nor, fortunately, the already-scarred knuckle that had borne the brunt of the force, such as it was. It never crossed my mind that a show of force would elicit anything other than hushed awe from a future wife: but wives are not middle-school boys.

Even when I *wanted* a story about knuckle-punching to come true, I couldn't find it in me to strike with conviction. Returning to my middle-school self, I remember a recurring dream—call it a nightmare—in which I was standing in the schoolyard, one hand handcuffed to my twin brother's. I would raise my other fist to punch him, but my arm would go frozen— paralyzed, useless. Night after night my arm would freeze in mid-punch. I know enough of Freud to read guilty aggression into that dreamscape. Whatever anger may harbor within me, *I have never let myself be a fighter.* I have absorbed punches over the years, but have not thrown one since childhood.

That sort of passivity is not food for storytelling if you're growing up male and blue-collar in the 1960s in Perth Amboy, New Jersey. But I've since learned that scars can tell other stories than adolescent masculinity. I'll get to these "other stories" shortly, but I'm not quite done writing about my father. If there was one thing that marked my youthful relationship with him (and that spilled over into my relationship with my brothers, my twin especially), it was a pervasive sense of rivalry. Our lives seemed more competition than collaboration, and my father was never above gloating when he'd beat one of his sons at a game or contest. I assume he was just "having fun," but the taunting angered me beyond words. Card playing was his modus operandi: he was a card sharp, and I could never beat him. So I studied chess and became, in time, a tournament expert. I was determined that he would never beat me in *something*, and that something was going to be chess. Once again, I'm aware of the Freudian-Oedipal symbolism: the declaration of check mate derives from the Persian *Shāh māt*, "the king is helpless." And I'm aware that, in becoming someone he couldn't conquer (at least in chess), I had become like him—though in my own game and in my own way.

Two summers ago, I visited my mother. We got out some old photos and found a picture of my father that I don't remember seeing before. It was an official navy portrait: he was a young man of nineteen, an enlistee after Pearl Harbor. What I did not expect to see was my own skinny nineteen-year-old face gazing back at me. All along, I thought he looked like my older brother, since he had grown heavy over the years and my older brother was himself of a naturally heavier build. But this photo of this late teenager was/is my father who was/is me. He wasn't wearing a monocle and he had no Schmiss. He didn't need one. And, I suppose, neither did/ do I.

Any time one reconsiders one's relationship with one's father, one revisits territories of the self. From this current distance, my adolescent fascination with the Schmiss seems a projection of Oedipal rivalry, aggression, and guilt rolled into one. Of course my father wasn't a Nazi; beyond his gloating gamesmanship, he was a man of few words and a strong work ethic. He had been hurt many times, too, at the soda plant and out on his delivery route. Once, while delivering a dolly full of soda cases, a floor broke underneath him and he found himself in the basement of a bar, his back broken. When I was in middle school, my emotional relationship with him alternated between rivalry and sympathy. As I reflect on my youth, I don't remember him hitting me. He insulted me profusely, and his words cut as bad as razors, but it's curious that I don't remember him hitting me. Did he break another man's arm, as the story goes? Probably no more than I "creamed a gypsy" with a knuckle sandwich. Yet it's a story that propped up his masculine image; it's the equivalent of a Schmiss, seemingly.

—————/—————

Dear Wilhelm,

My self-analysis is in fact the most essential thing I have at present and promises to become of the greatest value to me if it reaches its end. . . . If the analysis fulfills what I expect of it, I shall work on it systematically and then put it before you. . . . It is by no means easy. Being totally honest with oneself is a good exercise.

—Sigmund Freud, Letter (1897) to Wilhelm Fliess[1]

So here's what I've learned recently about the Schmiss and its history. Through the mid-nineteenth century to the end of World War II, the *Mensur* was a collegiate rite of passage predominant throughout Eastern Europe. Sword combatants would face each other at a prescribed distance, prepared to receive a "hit" or "smite" (hence the German Schmiss). Over time, protective eyewear and padded clothes were introduced, leaving only a portion of the body exposed—of which the cheek was prime real estate. Two physicians were to be in attendance, one for each combatant. One was not to flinch, but to show "stoic indifference" in receipt of his wound. The duel need not be long; and, rather than feared, an expert dueler like Skorzeny would likely have been sought after, given his swift and efficient delivery. Students lacking the will or the finances for membership in aristocratic clubs such as these were known to carve out their own Schmiss, often exaggerating the scar by opening the cut and filling it with horse hairs.

Among its nicknames, it was called a "bragging scar." Well, that's pretty much what I had made of my middle-school playground accident—my knuckle—no? While the notion of "stoic indifference" sounds nobler than the Nazism of my adolescent understanding, there's still vanity in the Schmiss. And this brings me to my final story.

I was a college undergraduate home for the summer. Reluctantly, I agreed to clean out the gutters of our carport roof. In the process, I caught my right shin against a piece of scrap aluminum. Rather than stanch the bleeding, I kept working and let the cut bleed until it congealed. I wanted someone—my mother in this case, since she had asked me to clean the gutters—to look at it, to bear witness to my stoic indifference in the performance of a distasteful task. I knew this attitude was petty, but I wanted a witness, nevertheless:

"Jim, your leg is bleeding."

"Oh, it's nothing..."

That fall, I returned to school in Washington, D.C., and I remember taking a bus that stopped at a VA hospital on its route. A young man about my age entered the bus. I assumed that he had just come from that hospital, since he was missing his right leg below the knee. It was 1974, by which time America had withdrawn its forces from Vietnam. But we had left traces. In the history that I fabricated for this young man, he had left his limb in a Vietnamese rice paddy. We sat across from each other and our eyes met, though he had already noticed that I had noticed his missing limb. I won't forget his look at that moment, though I lack words to describe it fully. There was a sadness in his eyes, but he gave a half-shrug and a grim almost-smile suggestive of embarrassment, as if to say, "I'm sorry. I'm sorry I lost my leg, and I'm sorry that you have to witness it." I may totally have misinterpreted, but this what I thought back then and I think it now, still. He neither wanted nor needed a witness for his too-real wound.

I've avoided war and am blessed for that fact. But what else, if anything, have I learned from this quasi-Freudian meditation? I should at least admit that my internal German-Polish conflict is a personal fiction: Baumlin is an Alsatian name, and Germany exchanged Alsace-Lorraine with France each time a war was won or lost. I may have no German blood whatsoever. I've learned to admire the Polish freedom fighters who stood, or fell, in self-defense. And while I admire many things German, I cannot in my adulthood admire the Schmiss. For all its collegiate ritualism, the Schmiss is itself a lie among battle scars—a masculinist prop, a piece of facial theatre, a show-off cut that mocks authentic wounding. Freud was right: "Being totally honest with oneself is a good exercise."

And I've learned not to tell stories about the origin and meaning of scars.

———/———

NOTES

1. "A single idea of general value dawned on me," Freud's letter continues. This "single idea" is the mythic rivalry with one's father, which he claims to "have found, in [his] own case too," and has come to "consider it a universal event in early childhood." It is here, in this early letter to Fliess, that Freud first articulates his theory of the Oedipus complex.

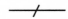

BIBLIOGRAPHY

Freud, Sigmund. "Group Psychology and the Analysis of the Ego." *The Standard Edition of the Complete Psychological Works of Sigmund Freud*, Vol. 8. London: Hogarth, 1985.

_____. *The Origins of Psychoanalysis. Letters to Wilhelm Fliess*, Drafts and Notes: 1887-1902. Edited by M. Bonaparte, A. Freud, and E. Kris. Translated by E. Mosbacher and J. Strachey. New York: Basic Books, 1954.

Quinodoz, Jean-Michel. *Reading Freud: A Chronological Exploration of Feud's Writings*. Translated by David Alcorn. East Sussex, UK: Routlege, 2005.

Rubin, Jeffrey B. "The Real Oedipal Complex." *Psychology Today Online*. May 1, 2012. Accessed March 31, 2014.

THE THOUSAND NATURAL SHOCKS
Chris Osmond

My scars are twinned: alopecia universalis for nearly twenty years, coupled with the traces of a dozen removals of dysplastic nevi over thirty.

Standing naked, the latter are drawn on the hairless canvas of the former, presence and absence, figure and ground. The scars are mostly shallow pits, round craters on the moonscape of my neck and abdomen. The dip between my shoulder blades holds a welter of angry snarls, though, poisonous pink rivers in a barren valley.

In brief: I am hairless as a guppy, and have had a lot of moles removed. One without the other would diminish the impact, but taken together they make me a formidable presence in the gym, at the pool. My sudden, hulking whiteness, the lack of eyebrows giving my eyes startling intimacy to yours may leave you uneasy about where and how my face emerges, or doesn't, at the peak.

The removal scars are prophylactic victories, successful assessments of my body as more or less likely to metastasize these little bumps into dragons that would swallow my sun. They are signatures of confident, preemptive action taken and could—should—be felt as such, touched with gratitude as dodged bullets that left a hole regardless. But they don't live that way, many days. To see this skin in the fogged mirror every morning is to remember and rewitness a series of microincursions into my physical and psychic integrity. They were night missions, hard-target searches that acquired their objectives and resealed the perimeter before anyone woke up.

But for all their remembered violence, the scars are not a referendum on my character. If anything, they celebrate my circumspectness: every six months to the dermatologist, see? (Perhaps I will die of nothing at all.) My alopecia, though, seems to have tons to say about who I am. When diagnosed, I was told it was caused by an autoimmune response triggered by a stress reaction, through which my system "shut down" my hair. Didn't "kill" it, the doctor was clear—the follicles "still work fine." They've just been bullied into submission, indefinitely, by an overreaching border patrol that regards them as suspect. In other words, my hairless skin marks me as someone who has been overwhelmed and hasn't gotten back up yet. Who doesn't get up when they are knocked down?

Moles scar by marking where they used to be, echoing the traumatic moment of their removal. Alopecia scars by marking where nothing is: what should be there is simply gone, echoing the traumatic moment of . . . what? I know what cut my skin. I don't know what shocked it. I'll see the blade coming, next time, maybe. But what else am I watching for?

Those are some of the mute questions my scars offer, daily. Here are some others: how was I cared for, in those settings where I was completely vulnerable to the incursions of those I trusted? How have I been written on by those long-forgotten interludes of trauma? What does my experience say to the thousand procedures that will be completed today in the rooms where I pursue my vocation, and my children theirs? Quite a bit, I think.

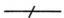

When I touch the scars where the nevi came off, I remember each procedure. Tiny studies in incongruity of unseen steel and ill-fit verbs. "We'll just punch it out," the dermatologist said when he did my back—and I thought of the shiny hole punch we'd use to confetti the cheap, grainy manila paper at school. I lay facedown on a table that does not recline flat, my back concave to improve access for the doc, becoming impossibly uncomfortable in order to offer myself up.

First the prick of the needle for the local, deeper than it should be and with it that sense of being pressed until you yield, no way to stop it: your will bending to its, here it comes, try to breathe. And the anesthetic ending the pain, certainly, but not the texture, the palpable substance of something happening back there, the way you can plug your nose to eliminate taste but not the feel of what's in your mouth. The shove and give, *Oh god you did what? Oh god.*

"Punch," for that one; "shave" was the word for the rest. Even after doing it a dozen times, I've never seen the blade. I imagined a good old Gillette disposable, but huge, big enough to accommodate the head of the mole, pass over and under it to dispose of it smoothly, goofproof. The first when I was thirteen. Just to the front of my left ear, a beauty mark, really, that caused no fuss until I started shaving and it would get nicked and irritated. That must be why I always pictured the daily razor, grown monstrous.

Punching and shaving. Never an actual cut, apparently, the word "cut" banned from these procedure rooms, the way "pain" becomes "pressure" in a dentist's office. Nipped-off bits, every year or so for a while there, leaving me leaking briefly, marked where the membrane that encases me was opened, then closed again. Echoes in each of the umbilical cut, in its dark little pocket—my primal divot, and yours, right there above our belts. A little thing, impossible to grok a time when that dead little pucker opened the whole wide freeway of life. But that one's shallow and bottomed on most of us, its depth and implications known, an ancient scar, no story we remember. These were pure and conscious wounds, opened surfaces encouraged to heal but never knit to how they used to be. Scar tissue being the only type of skin that only pulls one way, binding and twisting if coaxed against its artificial grain, itching, reminding.

Why did the cutting stop there, anyway? And what could I have done to resist had it not? When you are cut so deliberately, you wonder, at the ease with which your skin opened, how agreeably it would have yielded to a worse wound had the doc seen fit to persist. How absent any force to counter the blade. Echoes of circumcision, and the calculus my parents must have run before their consent: it's only outpatient, just a small thing really, more remarkable for its banality, don't mind his cries, don't cry. If we don't name them as cuts they won't hurt, but they did. Working through $2 draft night at the pool hall with friends after an abdominal removal, I used the word "gut shot" to describe how it felt. The beer not touching the pain as the anesthesia wore off.

A school is where they grind the grain of thought
And grind the children who must mind the thought

Howard Nemerov's lines, remembering the first day of school. That moment when the father releases his child for the first time to the institution that he knows will break her to remake her. He gets the logic, irrefutable. The grain must be ground for the germ to emerge, and the proliferation of what can be done with wheat justifies the violence, the mashing, the discarding of the stalk, the chaff, the husk, until only what is desirable remains. You'll be glad when this is over; wait till you see what you can do with what we've done to you.

School, though, wasn't a grinding for me. Great stretches of my natural form were left untroubled, for better or worse. No teacher ever raised a pen against my sentences, their length, perhaps, forbidding real incursion into how they might be broken down and better reconstituted. There's a whole stack of papers to grade, anyway—he's fine, A-plus. Literature class was simply a question of turning up the focus to meet the detail-obsession of any given teacher. Read for sense, or for the color of Daisy's sweater, the name of her haircut? I could suss that water easy enough, guide my boat between the rocks. A-plusplus, AP, go write, my child.

Math, I never even showed up: nothing above "cross-multiply-and-divide-it-out" even penetrated. A glimmer of sense in geometry—something about proofs, symmetry between two columns you could intuit and coax into being, lovely—but it blipped by in a semester, leaving me to the integers, the algorithms:

Three dozen bits and pieces of a stuff
So arbitrary, so peremptory,
That worlds invisible and visible
Bow down before it, as in Joseph's dream
The sheaves bowed down and then the stars bowed down
Before the dreaming of a little boy.

It didn't hurt because I wasn't there, really. Marking time and flirting with the teacher just to get through, then off to a liberal arts college that gave the gentleman a pass on any more of that quantitative stuff.

So no grinding for me; nothing so holistic, no complete dismantling. Thus, I was never reconstituted. What I'm baking with, if anything, is pretty much what I started with. I'm the same kid who started kindergarten, with three degrees and far better vocabulary.

But the punching and the shaving: plenty. After a particularly astute contribution to a third-grade discussion of the relationship of the permafrost to the tundra, Mrs. Perillo called me discreetly to her desk—to be congratulated on my erudition, no doubt. "Young man," she said sweetly, "do you know what 'pompous' means?" I did. And the screen goes black, what's said next forgotten in its sensation but not its texture, not its feel. Punch.

The year the alopecia happened, I took a group of high school students for a three-week home stay in Spain, and when my girlfriend picked me up at Dulles her first words were, "What happened to your eyebrow?" The dermatologist inspected the bald spot on the back of my head and the firebreaks in my leg hair (not from the new motorcycle boots, it turned out) and diagnosed me in less than a minute. "You'll probably lose it all within the year. No cure, but no further health concerns associated, nails might get brittle. See the nurse about treatment options." And he was gone, no doubt happy to have saved ten minutes in his afternoon schedule.

I lost the rest of my eyebrows pretty soon after that. My face without eyebrows was terrifying, alien. Even though it is impossible to really see yourself in the mirror the way others see you, I could sense that my expressions were off, skewed by their absence. My eyelashes must have gone about the same time, because suddenly there was gritty dust in my eyes. I never realized how useful they were until they were gone.

I kept losing hair. It came out in the shower over the next couple of months. I could feel my scalp under a light fringe at the back of my head, and knew I was looking progressively stranger. One day I decided that, if I was going to lose it anyway, I wanted to see what it looked like black, so I went to the drug store with my goth friends and bought a package of dye. The effect was ghastly, and I knew it: the pale of my weird featureless face all the more noticeable under bottle-black bangs.

Finally, I decided to bite off the inevitable and swallow the implications. I cut off the rest of my hair in the bathroom, then used an electric razor out on the deck to shave down the rest. It hurt to do it—I think the razor was dull—and it took a long time, much longer than I thought, with the Depeche Mode song "Clean" on an endless loop in my head. When I was done, I wet-shaved the whole thing carefully, trying to navigate the unfamiliar topography of my skull with the aid of two mirrors and some cursing. And then I was totally bald.

The first thing I noticed was the daily cold. I was cold, all the time, regardless of the weather. And the vulnerability—I ducked every time anything grazed my head, the slightest breeze magnified by nerve endings that had learned to ignore hair, but not wind. I seemed to experience air and light completely unmediated, as if for the first time. Ceilings seemed lower, the whole world newly sharp and right at eye level, where it stays to this day.

All from a "stress reaction." But what was the stress? Was I "punched" somewhere that made me lose my hair? Could it have been those nasty black Ducados I smoked in Spain like an ancient *pensionista*? ("Fumas mucho!" commented the school principal who was hosting me in his home as I came in from my pre-breakfast fix. When a Spaniard says you are smoking a lot, you are smoking a lot.) Maybe it was the crazy-strong strawberry brandy one of the host teachers made in his *pueblo* that had been passed around in an unlabeled bottle one night. God knows what was in that stuff.

Almost twenty years on, the alopecia is still unreadable to me, written clearly but in a language I don't know. Or perhaps I just know it too well to hear it told. Something chronic, perhaps, environmental? The toxic religion I was raised in and the sequelae of extracting myself? Internecine conflict, the ache of a ruptured self-image, phantom limbs, daddy issues, *ach du*? Perhaps I can discern it in the habits of constant vigilance I've developed: compulsive counting and concern for symmetry that rumbles deep in my lizard brain, obsession with arbitrary indicators of security and safety (milk in the fridge, dishes done, my keys exactly where I left them). Cause and explanation recede from me: no differential offered, action contraindicated in absence of more data. In southern emergency departments, a patient whose symptoms of being overwhelmed have inscrutable etiology is sometimes diagnosed as, simply, "DFO:" "Done Fell Out." So did my hair, and maybe so did I—for reasons unclear at present and, maybe, forever.

But it does murmur something about how contingent our integrity is upon factors we don't even know to check. How delicate our physical and emotional equilibrium is, how completely our alignment can be skewed by potholes we never see coming. How the infinite ways we might be hurt overwhelm our capacity for vigilance against them; that the only sanity is in reconciling ourselves to the bumps in the road and living in gratitude that we get to be on the journey at all. But this doesn't satisfy, not completely. I stubbornly think we can do better than reconciling ourselves to the thousand natural shocks. But there's no clarity there, yet.

What is clear is how my alopecia diagnosis and treatment story vividly echoes the themes of my nevi removals. The marks of presence and absence on my skin should represent care given and gratefully received, but they do not. They remind instead of little wounds inflicted by people doing their jobs a little less attentively than they should have. Therefore my scars signify not victory over death—caution exercised, life valued and saved— but carelessness, distractedness, pro forma responses, pain indifferently dished out and sewn up. Casual, sterile cruelty, easily and abundantly dispensed. We learn to live with it, of course, most intimately in our outpatient clinics and our classrooms, because we must. We must learn that the world is casually cruel, even when it's working for our welfare.

My scar stories do not lead me to argue against clean removal of dangerous moles, efficient diagnosis of chronic conditions, or correction of pompous students, of course. Rather, they indicate the primary need for care in the doing of those essential things: unfailing attention to how our words and our cuts land. A few minutes sitting with someone while they take in a life-changing diagnosis or devastating character assessment, and a moment of reset and recovery allowed after. We would still have the scars then, wouldn't we: would still be marked by the inexorable, necessary corrections. But then they would name people and faces, gentle hands and words, which held us as we suffered and, almost simultaneously, began to heal.

What do caring professionals need to be able to provide such care? Time to find their own peaceful, sustainable engagement with their vocations. Respect for the humanistic aspects of their labor, not just the measurable outcomes of their replicable "best practices." Space to discover the deeper wells of their capacity to notice, empathize, and act authentically in what Dan Liston calls the "suspended moments of living hope": ". . . we reach out with others to understand the texts we read and the lives we lead. We attempt to come to understand the many meanings before us, we reach for those meanings and, in reaching, we show features of ourselves. In reaching for those meanings we are attempting to bridge what we know with what we do not know, what is present with what is lacking."

I once heard the CEO of an academic medical center justify aggressive collection of unpaid bills by insisting "no margin, no mission." Caring professionals need margin to work with too, the better to answer the call for these uncompensated aspects of caring. Though such surplus is hard to reckon in quality assessment, its absence certainly is not. We simply cannot afford to leave it out of our figuring.

Maybe it's the constant stress of institutional work that makes the scars of failed healing more visible and painful. Upon the ground of chronic, low-level shock in which so many practitioners work, we can easily figure the wounds caused by inadequate efforts to heal, the marks of how incompletely the wounds have closed and knit. They pop, perhaps, against the unceasing backdrop of churning overwhelm, a signal against the noise.

Maybe this account makes a virtue of necessity, finding some scant value in failure. But if it weren't for my alopecia, I wouldn't see my scars as brightly; wouldn't be able to learn their lessons and advocate for better care the next time I go under the dermatologist's blade. I can trace the stories of my traumas more clearly when I can *see* them. Might those who work in caring professions do the same, "leaning in" to the stressors of the work instead of fleeing and fearing them, the better to articulate the damage our healing can cause? Paradoxically, perhaps we grow our capacity for empathy not by hoarding our energy, but by spending it freely: giving to receive, embracing the unpredictability of the clinical encounter and navigating it on its own terms, not ours. On the ground of chaos, the figures resulting from our efforts are more clearly drawn, and we can better decide what to do differently next time.

———/———

My scars are twinned: *alopecia universalis* for nearly twenty years, coupled with the traces of a dozen removals of *dysplastic nevi* over thirty.

Standing naked, the latter are drawn on the hairless canvas of the former, presence and absence, figure and ground. The scars trace the best efforts of a dozen physicians to help me, to save me: my hairless skin a dog-eared chart of all those workaday punchings and shavings. I read in them a cautionary story of how not to care for those entrusted to me, but also an account of people who have tried their best to lean in to the demands my body made on them by dint of their vocation. They chose to devote their lives to caring for me; I chose to ask them to.

The conditions in which we met were and are saturated by uncountable jolts and bumps, the thousand natural shocks that flesh is heir to. If we are compassionate and attentive, perhaps those very stresses can open our eyes to see the results of our actions, fit us to better meet the unfathomable depths of the world's need the next time we are called to try. As we live into our lives and our vocations, so are we revealed to ourselves, and to each other.

$$\underline{\hspace{2em}}\!\!\!\!/\underline{\hspace{2em}}$$

NOTES

1. "The Thousand Natural Shocks" was the winner of our 2013 Et Alia Press Scar Anthology Contest.
2. Liston.
3. This is not my idea; see the discussion of "exquisite empathy" in Kearney, et al.

BIBLIOGRAPHY

Kearney, et al. "Self-Care for Physicians Caring for Patients at the End of Life: 'Being Connected . . . A Key to My Survival.'" *JAMA* 301, Issue 11 (2009): 1155–1164.

Liston, Daniel P. "Love and Despair in Teaching." *Educational Theory 50*, Issue 1 (March 2000): 81–102.

Nimerov, Howard. "September, The First Day of School." *The New Yorker*, September 19, 1970.

$$\underline{\hspace{2em}}\!\!\!\!/\underline{\hspace{2em}}$$

THE POETRY OF MISCHANCE

Scott Huler

Have I shown you my fencing scar?

My wife rolls her eyes. She has heard it before. I angle my shoulders away. I am talking to you now. Kindly direct your attention here, at my finger, the middle one on my right hand—my foil hand.

"It is not a fencing scar!" June shouts. "A dog bit you!" But I am telling you a story; listen only to me, please.

Long and narrow, my fencing—quiet!—my fencing scar runs along the middle phalange, from the joint just below the tip to the joint at its base. Slightly ragged, the scar is hypertrophic. My body created a little more collagen than skin repair required, leaving the subject of our discussion: a scar. Significantly more collagen and you get keloid scarring, which spreads beyond the wound. Just the right amount and you get little more than new skin and nothing to show for your wound: simple healing, which is great, but nothing to show off.

That is, when the injury is small, our bodies simply resolve it; when the injury is larger or takes longer to heal, we end up with more than just healing. We get a monument. And, often, a story.

A scar is a story our body tells the world.

Like my fencing scar. Which does, to be honest, have rather a significant dog bite element to it, but, here: you be the judge.

In my sophomore year of college I signed up to take fencing, which satisfied somehow my image of the person I was trying to create. As a freshman I had taken calculus—I'm almost sure I called it "the calculus," thus: "Reasonable men and women ought to know the calculus." I make no apologies; I was a freshman in college. In the same way, knowing how to fence seemed like a way to help construct the dashing profile I planned to cut.

But funny enough, I seemed to have a flair for the foil. I commonly won our little class tournaments, and the instructor—the university's fencing coach, a former Olympian—urged me to join the team. Which, I suspect, ticked off whatever mastery goals I had for fencing. Not prepared to complicate my life with such commitments, I simply enjoyed the image of myself, practicing my doubles and parry quartes while some professor ran laps around the gym, always—always—playing a tape of the second movement of Beethoven's Seventh.

227

And to that soundtrack I did learn to fence. As beginners we focused almost exclusively on foil, and I learned to balance my weapon, as one did, on the ball of the first joint on my index finger, using my thumb to hold lightly, and to control the point—tiny, fine-motor movements describing swift arcs and spirals of the button at the end of the blade. To hold a foil as tightly as even a guitar pick makes for a hamhanded style, so to foster that gentle, balanced grip I eschewed the glove many fencers wore. An affectation, but again: I was winning class tournaments, so it didn't appear to harm my fencing—though because much beginning fencing involves less fine-motor surgery than wide, wild swipes, the fingers of my right hand commonly absorbed scrapes or even cuts.

Enter Fritzie, Patty Young's big black wire-haired terrier. On spring break I stopped on a jog to visit Patty, who wasn't home. On a whim I went around back, where I encountered Fritzie, behind the chainlink fence. No dog person, I nonetheless found in Fritzie the first of my lifelong series of dog companions. When we smoked pot in Patty's basement, Fritzie followed me around. Fritzie leaned against me during conversations, begged for my attention despite my evident lack of interest. So seeing her in the yard, feeling expansive, responding to her excitement and wagging tail, I greeted Fritzie and stuck my fingers through the fence to pat her. At which point she nonchalantly, even cheerfully, lunged and bit me, tearing a long, ragged gash along my middle finger and a similar, smaller one on the fourth. It surfaced later that Patty's brother's friends had used to tease Fritzie by poking her with sticks through that fence.

I commenced jogging with something of a purpose, ending up at my mother's place of work, expecting to borrow the car to drive to the hospital. This my mother proclaimed absurd, scolding me for my panic and telling me to run along home, wash my cut, and stop sticking my fingers through fences at dogs. Which I did—I did both—and watched the finger swell for two days before I did go to the emergency room, where a frowning doctor soaked my hand, cleaned the wound, and treated me like a brain-damaged child for having failed to come immediately.

The cut had barely begun to heal when, back at school, my first fencing opponent ripped it back open with a blind swipe. A day of healing, then back to fencing, and more insults to the healing skin. And again, and again, until finally I did put on that glove, though by then the damage was done, and what surely would have been at least a small scar under any circumstances had become a ridge of collagen, a mountain range bisecting the plain of my digit. Would you like to see?

So you tell me: fencing scar? Dog bite? Monument to foolishly delayed medical care? College boy fantasy? I tell you the story I like; with the scar my body announces it has a story to tell. The story is the book; the scar the cover art by which you are forbidden to judge it.

A scar is an item in the table of contents. The men in the boat in *Jaws* read their scars as litany, lovingly caressing them, reciting their stories trancelike: their scars are the traces their lives have left on their bodies.

Consider my track and field scar, which not only exists, but actually has the origin I claim for it. In the 8th grade track championship Bobby Fredrickson and I fought side-by-side for the lead in the 220 yard dash. Somehow legs became entangled and down I went, landing—and skidding for some distance—on hands and knees on the black cinder track. I remember running, with the finish line in view down the straightaway, then a jiggle to the camera of memory, and then I am standing, bent over, hands on thighs, blood running down both knees and both palms. A ninth-grader came over, wide-eyed, and guided me to the nurse's office, where I waited for my mom (who was significantly more understanding in my early adolescence than she would be six years later with Fritzie).

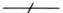

At the ER stitches were not possible. My right knee was a raw hamburger someone had dropped on the ground. A doctor numbed me with four shots of Novocaine and under a lamp picked out cinders with a tweezers and a magnifying glass, sending us on our way with dressings and lotion. For a day or two I pantomimed anger at Bobby Fredrickson, though I knew that the fall had been accidental. And though I enjoyed the celebrity of the incident and the accusations by those interested in fomenting conflict—"You were going to win until Bobby knocked you down!"—I never believed. My strength was drained on the curve at the beginning of the race; on the straightaway I flagged. I wasn't going to win. One quadrant of my right knee remains numb to this day, and a silver dollar-sized target of contoured skin tells the tale, as do tiny flecks of black in my knee and hands, remnants of that cinder track. The scar, apart from leaving a numb spot, is less supple than the skin around it, a perfect example of engineering at work: to gain strength, we sacrifice flexibility. This may work effectively as metaphor, as well. When we have an emotional wound, we heal by telling and retelling the story; to repair a physical wound we use a scar to join rent tissue. A scar is a story of another kind.

Of the tiny scar on my chin I can tell you only that I don't remember
it happening. I don't even remember the story except to say I've got it
conflated with the story of how when I was two years old our neighbor
swung open our back door just as I happened to emerge from the basement
stairs and sent me tumbling down, like Jack; also like him, I broke my
crown. The story is that I sat patiently perusing a book while the doctor
sewed up my head. Now that I think of it, another doctor similarly sewed
up my head decades later. The night before a backpacking adventure was
to start I bounded around a hotel room so gleefully that I bounded the top
of my skull right into a shelf corner. The shelf was metal; my cranium was
nearly as hard. Not so my scalp, which got the worst of it.

"You guys!" I shouted to my friends. "I fucked up! I banged my dome!
Come in for a second!" as I bled into a thin, scratchy towel, on which my
blood would scarcely leave the first stain. "Check it out," I said, moving the
towel. "I'm a dope, but it's okay, right?" They resounded in unison. "Sure,
let's see; you'll be . . . oh. Oh. We'd better call 911." Quitting our tiny motel
on winding mountain roads, we had to flag down the ambulance. The guys
in the truck recognized a hole they couldn't darn themselves and sent me
to the ER, where a pleasant young doctor sewed me up while I patiently
perused a magazine. We had to stop again a hundred miles up the trail so
someone else could cut the stitches out and replace them, as I understand
it, with glue. I taped the stitches on postcards and sent them to friends at
home: "Look!" My hair would cover the actual scar; the stitches were like
the mold the scar used as it set: the scar of the scar.

Or look at the narrow, two-stitch line that runs beneath my chin. I no
longer remember how I got it, but I suspect it was not unlike the way my
six-year-old, Gussie, got his, when at one-and-a-half he slipped on wet
kitchen linoleum, went down faster than you would think a little boy
could fall, and commenced yowling and bleeding from the chin with
equal intensity. As ER crises go it never got past code yellow. June had just
finished preparing dinner, and my mother-in-law happened to be over;
a nurse, she quickly corroborated our judgment that we needed to take a
drive. But no bit tongue, no soreness in jaw or anywhere else, and grandma
at home feeding the older brother removed much of the anxiety from the
trip, if not the trauma. "Oh, I know," we would say to Gussie in those days
when he cried and told of his injuries, so he had developed the habit of
sorrowfully moaning those words when he was truly hurt. So as the doctor
sewed on Gussie's Novocained chin and June and I helped the nurse hold
him down, he knew how to express his pain: "I know," he sobbed. "I know."

One day he will tell that story as some lover, head in his lap, looks up at his chin and traces a finger over that little scar. As lovers have done to the one on mine.

A scar is a story, and a scar is gentle. A scar seeks to heal the wound, not attack its cause.

And how after all, in our oldest tale, does the aged nurse Eurycleia, alone among those who have remained in Ithaca, recognize Odysseus, returned after twenty years, not only utterly changed but in disguise? By his scar. Not the scars of the Trojan War, which would have been a decade old and older, though still new to Eurycleia; and not the even newer scars he had won battling Circe, Scylla, and Poseidon on his way home. As she washes his feet, Eurycleia recognizes the scar on his thigh from a gash Odysseus received during his first wild boar hunt as a boy. Odysseus bore the scars of his earliest injuries, as do we all.

And Homer reminds us of the joy we get from those scars. "As for us, we'll sit here eating and drinking and recalling delightful old stories of our grievous misfortunes," he has the loyal swineherd Eumaus say to Odysseus. "It can be very sweet for a man whose wanderings and woes have been many to remember the hardships he had in earlier days." Which, if it's not that scene from *Jaws*, is at least its progenitor.

About our scars we have a great deal to tell; about our scars we could speak all day. Whether it's around a campfire in ancient Greece, at a galley table in a boat, in a cramped dorm lounge, or surrounded by loved ones calling foul on our exaggerations, our scars do what our stories do. They protect us. After all, after that dog bite in college I could have just worn the fencing glove and solved the whole problem, but what would I have to show for it? The scar turned a dog bite into identity.

And in the end, the story is worth the scar.

———/———

THOUGHTS ON VIOLET, THE MUSICAL

Stephen McNamee

Violet sets to music the story of Violet (Sutton Foster), who dreams of a miraculous transformation of a facial scar from a childhood accident. Convinced that a televangelist in Oklahoma can heal her, she boards a bus heading west. Along the way, Violet forms unlikely relationships with fellow riders which reveal lessons of beauty, love, and courage.

Part of me wished the musical took place in Scarsdale or Scarborough with the slogan being "Scarpe Diem" and with everyone wearing scarves while they scarfed down food and rode on scarnival rides that were set up near an escarpment. But the musical went in a different direction since the director, Leigh Silverman, decided against giving Violet a visible scar. Thus, the audience was required to imagine Violet's invisible scar in order to accept there was a scar the other characters couldn't see past.

Did Silverman elect not to mark Violet with a visible scar because she worried that if the audience was focused on the scar, we would be distracted from the other characters' inability to get past her disfigurement? This question actually confirms part of the sadness the musical captures. We all carry scars in one form or another, and yet, we don't permit those with the most visible scars forget about them as our lingering eyes and saddened facial expressions consistently remind the bearer of them. And yet, it's ironic that perhaps the only way to see beyond a person's scar is to truly acknowledge it—to stare it into normalcy. When the spotlight is fully on a person's scar (like in the musical, *Violet*), we cannot help but root for the scarred person, accept the scarred person, and see beyond her scar. This makes sense, since we all seek acceptance of and forgiveness for our own scars.

As the audience cheered for Violet during the musical, my eyes at times drifted away from the stage and to my fellow theatergoers. I wondered about the scars for which we were seeking acceptance. I wondered what scars we had created for which we were seeking atonement. As noted in the musical numerous times, we create new scars for ourselves and others every day, simply by using a poor choice of words, making a poor decision, choosing selfishness over selflessness.

However, watching the audience members and the musical's characters connect with Violet, it became clear that we are the solution as much as the problem. For all scars, the panacea is always the same—acceptance and forgiveness. Those are the only powers we have over scars. Those are the only powers we need over scars. Then again, *Violet* also made one other thing clear—those powers are hella more fun to witness and use while singing song after beautiful song.

———/———

Editor's note: Viewed by the author on Thursday, August 7, 2014 at the American Airlines Theatre in New York, New York, *Violet* is a musical by Brian Crawley and Jeanine Tesori, based on the short story "The Ugliest Pilgrim" (1973) by Doris Betts. "The Ugliest Pilgrim" was also made into a short film, "Violet," which won an Academy Award in 1981, and an earlier Off Broadway musical of the same name, which won a New York Drama Critics' Circle Award in 1998.

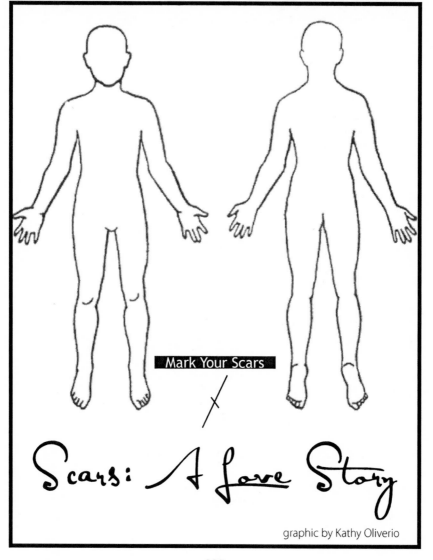

graphic by Kathy Oliverio

Scars: A Love Story

Jim Ferris

Scars

Scars are like ocean waves, but dried –
and pearly too – mountains who have tipped
their caps and now can't remember when
or why – or who – comets that always manage
to come by, rockets that jettisoned
stage one and two but press on,
no memory of ignition,
earnestly obedient to
trajectory, to thrust, to the
nameless being that remembers
simultaneously all things
and nothing (call it Santa Claus,
or God, or the electroweak
force), that which inures itself to
itself, that which takes every last
molecule of your body and
uses it for something else, if
not today, eventually.
Scar tissue is patience, and scars
ignorant mercy, memory
tough and carried on the skin.

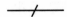

[Start slides of scar images . . . 300 different images, almost all in tight
closeup . . . give them a few minutes . . .]
Hi. How are you?

The Trouble with Poets [tuning: CGCFBbD] [song by Peter Mulvey]

The trouble with poets is they talk too much
They tell us it hurts them a little more
And we cannot tell if they make this up

We've never stood in their shoes, in skins, in their heads, on their shores
[...]
I think the trouble with poets is they see poetry everywhere

According to an article in the 326th volume of the British Medical
Journal,

> Each year in the developed world 100 million patients acquire scars, some of
> which cause considerable problems, as a result of 55 million elective operations
> and 25 million operations after trauma. There are an estimated 11 million keloid
> scars and four million burn scars, 70 percent of which occur in children. Global
> figures are unknown but doubtless much higher. People with abnormal skin
> scarring may face physical, aesthetic, psychological, and social consequences
> that may be associated with substantial emotional and financial costs.

Can you remember your body before life began to take its toll? Can you
imagine the body you inhabit right now without marks—without scars?

[look at slides a moment.]

How is it that you recognize yourself?

I have no memory of my body unscarred. I underwent my first surgery
on my first birthday, a lovely symmetry which is reflected in reverse, like
a photographic negative, in the radical differences between my legs, one
of which was the object of that and many subsequent surgical operations.
"Like a patient, etherized on a table . . ." The surgery does not deprive me of
the image of my young body unscarred . . . but it does take away any claim
I can make of that picture as memory.

[a few notes are played on the melodica . . .]

When was the last time your body was unscarred by this life? In your
mind, follow the contours of your body as it used to be. Start wherever you
like, your ankle, say, before you sprained it, your knee before you fell on the
gravel, your chin before that fall down the stairs.
   In your mind's eye, imagine a diagram of your body: head, neck,
shoulders, arms and trunk, hips, legs, feet. Does it look anything like the
diagram on your program? Now, using not only your mind's eye but also
your mind's magic marker, mark the location of your own scars. In fact, go

ahead and use a pen or pencil and mark them on the page. Be explicit, be
thorough—you don't have to show this to anyone . . . but do note them.

A mentor used to tell me not to judge it when I was in pain. It's a
sensation, that's all. Just notice it. Breathe into it. When you do this, pain
always changes. Try breathing into your scars right now. No judgment;
there is no way to do it wrong. Just breathe. As Heraclitus taught us long
ago, change is the only constant.

The opposite of scars is life unlived. How else can we tell ourselves apart?

Scars are places where the separation of inside and out has been
breeched and then reestablished. Scars help to keep outside out and inside
in. But they also mark that breech, even historicize it: a breech occurred
here . . . and it may return.

[a little more on the melodica]

Is it easier to imagine your front than your back? I know it is for me.
But there is such interesting architecture from that less imaginable angle,
dips and flares, bulges and creases. Is that really what the back of my
head looks like? It's like hearing your voice in a recording: is that what I
sound like? Really? When I taught public speaking years ago we had video
cameras mounted in the ceiling to record student speeches. I remember
getting ready for class one day, setting up the camera, just comping the
shot, focusing and such. The shot caught the back of my head, and I was
startled to see a bit of skin peeking through at my crown. Shining through,
more like. The video from the next class confirmed, just a little thinner
there. And soon I had turned it into a jokey little piece of performance: oh,
getting a little thin on top. Doing a Prince William impression, are we?

Suddenly that thinness became a short piece in my performance
repertoire. Perhaps I couldn't control those follicles, but I could do . . .
something with them. For years I couldn't to a thing with my hair: it was an
unruly bush that refused all my attempts to put it in its place. Now, though,
I could put it in its place, at least metaphorically. I couldn't control the hair,
but the perception of the hair—now that's another story.

Maybe. How much we actually get to control other people's perceptions
. . . From the Cleveland Clinic: "Remember this basic truth: scars never
completely go away." Unlike hair, I guess.

Scar tissue forms as the body's response to insult or injury. Scars are divots taken out of the fairways of our bodies, scars are pearls fused into flesh. Pearls grow in response to irritation—more insult than injury. Scars, on the other hand . . .

I have no memory of my body unscarred. The typo that I corrected here reads, "I have no memory of my body unscared." That, as Dr. Freud taught us, could be telling. But my earliest memories, I have no doubt, are fabrications. The picture of my mother holding the tiny me outside the hospital in the chill November air . . . Nice picture, but I see it from the perspective not of the little one in mother's arms but of one watching the scene. Does memory always have point of view? That picture is so clear in my mind. Where does it come from? My imagination? An old movie? I'm just not sure about the perspective-taking ability of that one-year-old.

Again from the *British Medical Journal*, a clinical review of skin scarring from Doctors Bayat, McGrouther, and Ferguson:

> Scars are the end point of the normal continuum of mammalian tissue repair. The ideal end point would be total regeneration, with the new tissue having the same structural, aesthetic, and functional attributes as the original uninjured skin. Scarless skin healing occurs in early mammalian embryos, and complete regeneration occurs in lower vertebrates, such as salamanders, and invertebrates.

They continue:

> What, if any, are the advantages of scarring, and why do we scar? We hypothesise that wound healing is evolutionarily optimized for speed of healing under dirty conditions, where a multiply redundant, compensating, rapid inflammatory response with overlapping cytokine and inflammatory cascades allows the wound to heal quickly to prevent infection and future wound breakdown. A scar therefore may be the price we pay for evolutionary survival after wounding.

These cytokines, by the way, are small proteins that trigger the body's inflammatory and immune system responses. What is it that triggers the stories that inevitably arise around scars?

At least a couple generations of scholars, philosophers, film critics and others who love to drink little cups of very strong coffee have made the point that we humans make sense of ourselves and the world around us through story. It doesn't seem like a radical or shocking notion to us, I suspect. I first encountered this idea in an explicit and more or less systematic way in Walter Fisher's narrative paradigm, which he contends does not so much counter the reigning rational world paradigm as subsume it. If we make sense of the world through story, then the logical argument of the rational world paradigm can be seen as one kind of story, and not the only kind or the best kind.

Fisher proposed thinking of our species as *homo narrans*, storying human, to name and claim that we are, at essence, storytellers.

[go up to someone in audience; shake hands]

Hi. How are you? [small talk for a moment]

We certainly narrate our bodies. Think of the stories parents tell of their babies . . . and their bodies . . . not only mom's narrative of labor and that transcendent moment when it all became worthwhile . . . but the sitting up crawling standing walking narration, vocalizing, teeth, and talking . . . and the fears and concern when the story goes off-track . . .

[go up to two or three more people. be sure to ask "how are you?"]

How are you? Standard greeting, right? And the responses I received just now were all socially appropriate responses, right? Standard greeting as opening gambit in a small-talk encounter. What scholars as different as Bronislaw Malinowski and Roman Jakobson would call phatic communication, which is usually explained as communication more about opening and maintaining a channel for social interaction than about the actual content . . .

[to another person] How are you?

But what if we took that standard greeting as an invitation to narration? An invitation to narrate about how you are in the moment: body, psyche . . . relationally . . . financially . . .

[to another person] How are you?

The body has so many ways to remember, so many kinds of memory. There are scars, certainly, but also calluses, muscle tone (or the lack thereof), the ways that we train our bodies with clothes, with belts and brassieres. Not to mention the thing we call memory itself, which is surely bodily, not only in storage process and location, but also in . . . outcome? Maybe.

[melodica]

Performance is ephemeral, is an evanescent thing, while scars are
an imperfect record, a mark of a particular moment. We do all sorts of
things to record and fix moments of our lives: scrapbooks and keepsakes,
photographs and recordings both audio and video. And these records
always leave something out.

The records we make always come unmoored in history, in story, maybe
even in time . . . Alzheimer's is the great and scary unmooring, maybe
especially to academics . . . but perhaps the unmooring is inevitable. Think
of photographs from an earlier time . . . let's say 1970 . . . for some of us,
that is an eternity ago, ancient history, long enough ago that we weren't
even born yet, too long ago to even quite comprehend . . . while for others
of us, it is more or less recent history, a time we experienced and remember
. . . sort of . . . hair styles, fashions and passions of a different time. Not all
that different, perhaps, but think of trying to explain 1970 to an eleven-
year-old . . . before texting, before cell phones even, before the Internet,
back when a computer filled a big air-conditioned room with raised floors .
. . you used punch cards to connect with this enormous computer . . . nerdy
guys with pocket protectors hanging around. Okay, so some things don't
change that much, but now sometimes nerdy is cool, now nerdy women
may be in those rooms as well, and you don't see many pocket protectors
anymore . . .

[melodica]

At an estate sale a couple years ago I picked up an envelope of
photographic negatives . . . I'm not really sure what led me to buy them
. . . family photos of a family that is now gone. Or at least dispersed . . .
Snapshots of moments no one any longer knows . . . unmoored . . .

Scars can moor memory, at least to a specific place on the body that was
. . . I have a scar on my right thumb, it starts near the corner of the nail—
my nail—and runs down across the fleshy part around to the other side
at the first joint . . . it's been there so long I seldom even notice it . . . but
when I bump my thumb in just the right place, it feels like just the wrong
place, and boy do I remember it. I got that scar when I was three? Four?
Five? Mom was using a meat grinder, one of those hand-crank grinders—
before food processors—and I wanted to help. So I pushed the meat down,
and almost cut off my little-boy thumb. Fortunately, the doctor at the
emergency room was able to stitch me back together . . . and I've been
vegetarian for many years . . . not related to an event the specifics of which
I recall through other people's stories, especially my mother's . . . but when

I whack my thumb in that place I re-member, I re-embody that event and the way it changed my body all these years later . . .

A few years ago I asked my mother about that thumb-in-the-meat-grinder incident . . . she scarcely remembered it . . . we were living in Maywood at the time, a working-class suburb about ten miles due west of Chicago's Loop . . . I was still in a high chair . . . she was grinding up cranberries for cranberry relish . . . and it was my brother Bill who turned the grinder crank which nearly cut off my thumb . . . I'm still vegetarian, whatever the food in there was . . . but now I have something new to blame my brother for . . .

[melodica]

Here's a funny thing: that injury to my thumb has been healed for decades—but I still have a scar from it, and I still have the altered nerve from it . . . a breech occurred here . . .

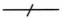

It used to be common knowledge that our bodies are constantly in regeneration mode, replacing cells left and right so fast that no cell in your body is more than seven years old . . . So much of what we know, we don't know. Carbon-14 dating, particularly the work of Dr. Jonas Frisen at the Karolinska Institute in Sweden, shows that some cells—neurons in the cerebral cortex, for example—are never replaced, they are with us for life. Others are replaced at faster or slower rates. How exactly that keeps this scar in place—it seems likely that all those cells have been replaced a number of times, but in that replacement process the scar is rebuilt in just the same place, it looks and feels like it did twenty or even thirty years ago. How exactly that happens is a mystery to me—though I'll bet someone can explain it.

[Music: melodica? song?]

I know a guy, he must own twenty-five different canes. Most of them are in a big crock in his living room, but he told me he's thinking about putting three or four in each room so that when he's not wearing his brace—he wears a brace kind of like mine to help him walk—but when he's not wearing it he can just pick up a cane in whatever room he's in and leave it in whatever room he goes to . . . figuring that whatever room he would leave, well, he would have to go into it first, right? So the number of canes in each room at any time might be vary somewhat, but on balance they should average out, right?

This guy—it's actually me, but if I talk about myself in the third person, maybe it's more of a story. D'ya think? I get so tired of the first person sometimes.

[melodica]

This is just a weird thing to do a show about, no matter how performance art-y or narrative-y, how post-modern, post-human, even post-contemporary it is. Scars are sites of wounding, sites of pain and suffering, even when they are more or less chosen, like in ritual scarring, like in branding, like in self-cutting.

[watch scar images for a moment]

I feel enormous gratitude to the many people who have shared their scars, their bodies, with me. What an intimate act, opening up to give of themselves, to give me their scars . . .

The burn scars are the hardest for me to look at—I think because they look the most painful, the broadest, the tightest. The most shocking. I heard a story on the radio a while back about people caught in the eruption of Mount Merapi, the volcano in Indonesia: the gases were so hot that in some cases they fused clothes and even mattresses to people's skin.

Burn scars look most likely to contract, too. "The natural history of scars," a plastic surgeon told me, is that "all scars want to contract." Which can be a problem, to say the least.

But not to look, to overlook, to look away, to participate in the erasure of the experience the scars represent—can you erase someone's scars without erasing them? Is over-looking a kind of overlooking? Overlook has at least a couple senses: to over-look, to look and look and focus so much on scars that all you see is the scars—and perhaps yourself—and not the person; and to overlook, to not see, to not notice, to look past . . . In either of those cases, the scars become another occasion for loss.

I wonder if the only thing worse than looking . . . is not looking.

Because scars may be sites of wounding, of pain, of suffering. But they are also distinguishing marks, signs of strength as well as vulnerability, sites of the body reclaiming, re-asserting its integrity in the face of injury. As a stem-cell therapy scientist who saw an earlier incarnation of this performance told me, scars are stronger than what was there before them . .

. maybe less flexible, maybe less cute, but stronger . . . And this applies even when the wounding is intentional, like in cutting. Like in surgery.

But what about when the surgeon makes a mistake?

And what about scars beneath the skin? I wonder.

[watch scars again]

I first heard of this in relation to a sort of initiation ritual at a fraternity at a historically black men's college . . . the young men would brand each others' skin with a coat hanger or some other hot object . . . I was shocked, and I don't think I shock easily . . . it seemed so painful, so dangerous and atavistic . . . it's since been copied by white fraternities . . .

And maybe it's a way of claiming one's body: I will scar myself before the world can . . . I get to assert what this mark means . . . it's a little more extreme than reclaiming a word like *queer* or *crip* . . .

[a little music]

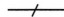

Is it true that different colors of skin scar differently? Race and the contested past, race and the ever-contested present . . . the scar on the Americas that surely has not faded . . .

Who is your tribe, your clan, your family? How do you know them? After a performance of this show, a man named Dannabang who grew up in Ghana told me about the marks that people commonly bear in West Africa. They are not scars, he said, these are not wounds but signs, assertions of identity. There are different marks indicating each tribe; and within the tribe, each clan; and within the clan each family. Your marks tell who you are. By your marks may strangers know you.

Dannabang told me about a fellow West African he came to know in Toronto. The man was upset at how he was repeatedly mocked for the marks on his face while in medical school. This was a proud man, from a prominent clan and a noted family, and the insults from the ignorant Canadians wounded him deeply. He decided to take the radical step of having his facial marks—his identity—removed through plastic surgery. The plastic surgery did not go well, and left the man with neither the smooth face that was prized in Canada nor the marks of his identity when he went home to West Africa to practice medicine.

Who is your tribe, your clan, your family? I feel for this man, who doesn't quite fit in either world. I recognize him as one of my tribe . . .

[melodica]

Do we become habituated to scars? I certainly am to mine. They become just a part of the landscape of the body . . . a little more flesh than I'd like here . . . a divot there . . . And scars fade over time, at least many of them do. Perhaps, they stop signifying, too. Perhaps, they're just there, perhaps they don't mean, they just exist with us . . .

Nah. But it does bring up that whole question of how meaning arises, whether it inheres or whether it is always attributed, always a social production, like communication it's not there until it is pronounced . . . at least in some way . . . like speaking the names of god to evoke the divine presence . . .

The scar is such a readily available metaphor: a scar upon the land, scarring the night sky, scarred for life. The tsunami scarred the coastline and miles inland . . .

But doesn't taking scar as metaphor obscure if not obviate real scars? I don't want real experience and real people overlooked so that we can toss scars around as metaphors . . . wait: that's a metaphor. Lots of great thinkers, I.A. Richards and Wittgenstein to name just a couple, tell us that there is no language without metaphor . . . but it pains me to commit metaphor when the price is so high. Forgive me – I know not how else to speak . . .

———/———

"What does not kill me makes me stronger." I think people believe that . . . some people, anyway . . . it puts me in mind of my mother, who dealt with pancreatic cancer for three and a half years before she left us a couple years ago . . . she had the famous Whipple procedure—a pancreaticoduodenectomy—a really long and hairy surgery removing all or part of the pancreas, gall bladder, stomach, duodenum, common bile duct, and more. She must have had a serious scar from that . . . I never saw it, never really wanted to . . .

And then I wonder if she saw all of my scars. All the early ones, I'm sure—including that thumb. But later ones? . . . and then there are scars that one cannot see without looking quite closely . . . scars that no one can see . . .

Got any of those?

What is a scar, exactly . . . My *Dorland's Illustrated Medical Dictionary*, 23rd edition, defines "scar", from the Greek eschara, as "cicatrix." Period. OK, cicatrix—which is pretty much Latin for ... scar. But let's look "cicatrix" up. Aha! "A scar." But wait—there's more: "the new tissue which is formed in the healing of a wound." The entry goes on to define a number of kinds of cicatrices:

> *filtering*, "a cicatrix following glaucoma operation through which the aqueous humor escapes"—and that's surely not funny;

> *hypertrophic*, "a hard, rigid tumor formed by hypertrophy of the tissue of a cicatrix." Wait a minute: don't they know you're not supposed to define a word by using the word? Come on. At least give us a word which means the same thing in another language. 'Cause that's useful. *manometric*, "a cicatrix of the eardrum that moves in and out with variations of the intratympanic pressure";

> *vibratory*, "which moves with the pulse, the respiration, or the voice";

And my favorite, *vicious*, "a cicatrix which causes deformity or impairs the function of a part." The word vicious by itself the dictionary defines as "1. Faulty or defective; malformed. 2. Depraved; refractory or unruly."

To be fair, my copy of Dorland's was published in 1957. And I didn't want to pay the $51 it would cost to get the 31st edition – even though that also includes access to the online version of the dictionary . . .

[play a little music]

Scars are the past, surely, signs of the past, physical and visual memory, yes, but they are also the present, the body's response to injury, the body's bridge. Are they as well the future? They are at least a future: how would we hold ourselves—our stories—together without our scars?

Is it fair to say our first scar, the one we all share, the mark of original sin, is our navel, the bellybutton, the umibilicus—or do you say UM-bul-I-cus? I had a professor in college, who taught intellectual history: he had a

[in a ponderous voice]

strange predilection for overemphasizing the last sounds of words.

I remember him talking about an ancient scholar, one of those intellectual giants declared a Doctor of the Church – a Doctorr of-uh the Church-uh: Saint Jerome – or do you say JER-ummm. And I remember thinking, nobody says JER-umm (let alone JER-ummm-ahhh). But his style has stuck with me, and I keep thinking maybe I should try it, in the classroom—or do you say, clossroom-uh?

My Dorland's defines "navel" as . . . the umbilicus. So I page back to the U's . . . and there it is. Umbilicus: the cicatrix marking the site of attachment of the umbilical cord in the fetus. And by the way, for umbilical it says "pertaining to the umbilicus." I guess definitions, like life, have an inherently cyclical if not circular quality to them. But Dorland's says that this mark we all share is indeed a cicatrix, a scar. It is a scar which, according to *Mosby's Medical Dictionary*, (8th edition, accessed online) "interrupts the linea alba about halfway between the infrasternal notch and the pubic symphysis. It is located at the level of the interspace of the third and the fourth lumbar vertebrae."

The navel, the umbilicus, the omphalos. Is yours an innie or an outie? The vast majority of people have innies, because their navels are nailed right into the abdominal wall. I've heard it said that an outie is a sign of great courage or intelligence, I can't remember which . . . but I'm sure it was someone with an outie who told me . . .

Speaking of early scars . . . how many of the men here are circumcised? In all the thinking and reading I did to get ready for this performance, circumcision scars never once occurred to me . . . until a wise friend said, "Hey, how come you don't talk about circumcision scars? I was waiting for circumcision scars" . . . Another voluntary scar, though not perhaps always a happy one . . . Gives new meaning to the idea of voluntary, too, doesn't it, because it's probably not the infant's choice.

[A little more music]

How did you do using your big forebrains to mark the location of your scars? More than one person, when I asked them if they had any scars they would let me photograph, initially responded "Oh, I don't have any scars." And then after a moment, "You know what, actually . . ."

Which makes me think of the subterranean life of scars. Scars can be cutaneous and subcutaneous at the same time. It stands to reason that they might be both conscious and subconscious, strophe and antistrophe. The ways of the mind are mysterious, although neuroscience plumbs ever

farther the dim and dusty inner recesses that make us the complex and
vexing outworkings of all those little chromosomes when the air gets to
them. How does your brain work without oxygen? Can a glass of water
change your mind? Can you change your mind?

Nature and nurture, what God hath joined together let no knife put
asunder.

Enter the scar, the body's act of love for itself, part for part, bridging
what has come apart . . . or perhaps walling off injury or insult?

Is it necessary for us to love our scars if we are to truly love ourselves?
When you noted yours, did you identify which is your favorite?

In our talkback session following an earlier performance, a woman told
us that she didn't have any favorite scars . . . she didn't like her scars . . . and
she was disappointed to learn that, according to her faith tradition—which
I think is Catholic—she will still have her scars in the afterlife . . . Father
Jose said you keep your scars . . . I think the explanation was that Jesus had
his scars after the resurrection, so it would be fitting for his followers to
keep theirs too . . .

A friend who was raised Catholic told me that Jesus didn't have scars, he
had wounds . . . which would mean that they didn't ever heal . . .

So why did Jesus keep his scars or wounds after his body was perfected?
Saint Thomas Aquinas, another Doctorr of-uh the Church-uh, explained
them as "an everlasting trophy of his victory." Christ's followers, he
suggested, might keep their wounds and scars, which "Will not be a
deformity, but a dignity in them; and a kind of beauty will shine in them."

One of the things I initially thought I would be doing today is narrating
my own scars . . . the nickel tour of some of the incursions into this body
. . . and there is one that I would like to tell you about—I think it would
qualify as my favorite. It's on my left wrist. It's two and a quarter inches
long. The plastic surgeon I interviewed for this performance said "it's a very
good scar." And I would have to agree: it is neat and unobtrusive, it doesn't
call attention to itself, it does not restrict the motion of my wrist . . . but
what makes it my favorite scar is how I got it.

I was picking a grocery bag out of the trunk, for some reason holding
it out from my body, and suddenly—I don't know if I heard or only
imagined a popping sound—but my wrist started hurting . . . a lot. It took
a few weeks to figure out what the problem was . . . but a ligament holding
two bones in my wrist together, the scaphoid and the lunate bones, had
disrupted itself.

The good news is that I had quite successful surgery to reattach the ligament. Before I agreed to this surgery I had an extended conversation with the hand surgeon, Dr. Steve Zachary. I told him about my long and checkered surgical history, not just the pain and loneliness and the uncertainty—you never know just what's going to happen when you let somebody make you unconscious and then take a knife to you—but also the responses to general anesthesia, all the puking and puking and puking . . . He told me he would get the anesthesiologist who did the very best arm block, so I wouldn't even need a general.

On surgery day the anesthesiologist persuaded me that, with much advanced materials and techniques, he could give me a general without the horrible side effects. And he was right—that all went fine. But what was even more important was the surgeon: he was not just highly competent technically, he was so careful of me the person, not just me the wrist to fix. Checking in with me, explaining everything, answering every question I had, and I had plenty. Talking to me like I was a big boy, like I was not just a broken object to be fixed but a thinking, feeling person. Like I mattered.

After the surgery I told him how much I appreciated that, and he told me that shortly after his daughter was born she needed surgery. He said he'd never forget what it felt like to hand over his tiny little newborn daughter to the surgeon, even somebody he had confidence in. He told me that he remembers that experience each time before he starts an operation, and then he works in the ways that he wanted others to work on his daughter.

This is Steve Zachary's scar. And that's why it's my favorite.

A breech occurred here, but now it is healed. Imperfectly, imperfectly, but healed. I hope we'll have some time to talk afterward—if you'd like, perhaps you could tell about your favorite scar.

The great French poet Paul Valery said, "A poem is never finished, only abandoned." Our scars go on while we go on. And now it is time for us to go on.

———/———

NOTES

1. http://my.clevelandclinic.org/disorders/scarring/derm_overview. aspx
2. Bayat, et al., 88.
3. Ibid.
4. *Dorland's Illustrated Medical Dictionary*.

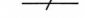

BIBLIOGRAPHY

Bayat, A., D.A. McGrouther, M.W.J. Ferguson. "Skin scarring." *British Medical Journal 326*, issue 7380 (January 11 2003): 88–92. Also available online at: http://www.ncbi.nlm.nih.gov/pmc/articles/ PMC1125033/.
Dorland's Illustrated Medical Dictionary, 23rd Edition. St. Louis: W.B. Sauders Co., 1957.

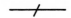

We Scar, We Heal, We Rise

Erin Wood

I imagine I am standing on the moon and there is the Grand Canyon below me. Someone has cleaved the Earth with a bowie knife and spread it wide to see what is inside.

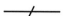

When they cut my thigh open to remove the infection, the doctor told me it would leave no scar, but eight weeks later it was clear that he was wrong. The day after the operation, the nurse stood at the edge of my hospital bed with her lips pinched together like a clam's shell. The morphine couldn't touch the feeling that my muscles were being pulled out along with the snake of gauze that she drew from the selvage of my skin and into her hands. After the first wretched session died down, I heard that my muscles were going to leave with the snake twice a day, every day, until my nerves sealed off and the glowing watermelon flesh locked back and there was nothing left but sutures and milky skin. When I had to change my own dressing, I learned that I have an impulse not to inflict pain on myself. This instinct is nearly impossible to overcome. After I fainted and came back in the shower, I looked into my leg like it was an oracle, but it told me nothing. Touching the guts of my thigh made me feel wicked, like yanking a turtle out of its shell and leaving it to rot.

In a photograph, my grandfather holds me tenderly with his pliant surgeon's fingers. I was a tiny, sick baby in a pink gingham dress with a bow Scotch-taped to my head. He was a man who had cut soldiers' arms and legs from their bodies with a saw three days after D-day. The soldiers' flesh was an envelope sealed up to keep the rest of them inside. The amputation saw he brought back from Omaha Beach was a token from the world that died behind him.

I have never *not* thought of my body in quarters. Across my belly, a barbed-wire path runs away from my center in four directions. It is a compass pointing toward others. It is a legend that shows them where I have been. Nine times doctors have opened me from the center to try to make me better, and in some ways I am. Until just before the last surgery, I only thought of what I could see on the outside, which was less than one side of the story. My topography can be flipped inside out to reveal reticulated growth that spreads slow and steady like a cantaloupe vine, commandeering other organs, holding them hostage, choking them off.

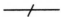

I have heard plenty about ghost limbs and I know that sensations can still act on the brain even when the eyes tell the brain that nothing is now where something used to be. It is too hard to believe an organ that has been around for thirty-three years would suddenly not be there anymore. But maybe when the ghost waits under skin and lymph and corpuscles, the eyes can't toy with the whole thing. We are always *not* used to our insides. When they are closed inside us, our organs are always reluctant phantasms; they have to be conjured up.

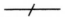

Whenever I have taken time to recuperate, I have noticed things I've never seen before. The last time I was ill, I saw a robin perched on my fence, panting in the heat. Now that I feel better, I let her open her beak inside me. Her breathing makes me feel alive.

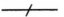

I read there is a museum in California full of medical curiosities. If you visited it, you would learn it was once thought that children could be cured of disorders of the mouth and throat by wrapping their lips around a duck's beak and drawing in its breath. You would learn that Medievalists believed eating ant eggs could cure the love-sick. You would be reminded that we need antidotes, and so we search.

I walked past a shady yard with trees so tall they hinted that I was nothing. The ground below them was a closely clipped carpet of green, some moss, some grass. Despite the mowers and the shadow of the canopy, an oak seedling found a place to grow inside a broken up drain pipe. Living things have a will to perpetuate.

Though it seems dangerous, to get hydrangeas to put on blooms you must prune them. Cut them where they v-off and they will pop off new blossoms within days. Bring the cut ones inside and, before you put them in water, burn their stems with a match. This way, they will live longer. Behind this violence lies a sort of kindness.

I told a yoga instructor that I was surprised when she called *savasana* the corpse pose. She looked at me as if she knew an awakening had escaped me and asked me if I feared death. Perhaps our misunderstanding is more a matter of perception. When she tells us to imagine we are melting into the earth, I picture myself hovering just above it.

Some things fly even though they don't have wings. When the larvae of the beach tiger beetle want to move on a windy day, they throttle themselves into the air to catch the breeze and become wheels clambering up dunes. With only one leap, they can move two hundred feet toward somewhere new.

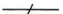

When my husband was eight, he was attacked by a Chow in his friend's front yard. It ripped his face open just below his lips on the left side and the dog kept lunging for him until it tore his arm down to the blue meat. I watch him as he strokes our hundred and thirty-eight pound Bullmastiff on the living room rug, both of them lying on their sides, staring at each other. My husband bends toward him and kisses him on his muzzle and coos in his ear until they both close their eyes.

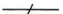

A scan of my middle would reveal a muscle man in my pelvis: A boxer, his gloves raised over his head like a champion without arms, his fists waiting to rise up and down in victory even though there is nothing to give them movement.

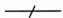

I imagine I am standing at the base of the Grand Canyon and there is the moon above me. The barbed marks of living are all around and all throughout me, opening and closing and shifting. Someone has exploded craters in the moon. Our celestial body has sealed them off. It shines.

About the Editor

Erin Wood writes and edits in Little Rock, Arkansas. Her essay "We Scar, We Heal, We Rise," was chosen as a notable essay in *The Best American Essays 2013*. Her essays have been read and broadcast on *Tales from the South*. Her essays, book reviews, fiction, and poetry have appeared on anderbo.com, and in *The Healing Muse, The Emprise Review*, and elsewhere. Wood owns and runs *Et Alia* Press with two partners, is a freelance professional writer, and teaches a course in literature and medicine at University of Arkansas for Medical Sciences. She has taught writing at Wrightsville Prison, The Clinton School of Public Service, and University of Arkansas at Little Rock. Wood received an A.B. in English from Duke University, a J.D. from Georgia State University College of Law, and an M.A. in professional and technical writing with a focus on nonfiction writing from University of Arkansas at Little Rock. She is currently writing a memoir about her family's experience in the Neonatal Intensive Care Unit. Learn more at https://erinwoodwritingandediting. wordpress.com.

———/———

Contributors

Bennett O'Brien Battle is a native of Little Rock, Arkansas. He received his BA in English from Tulane University and recently graduated medical school at the University of Arkansas for Medical Sciences. He is currently in his first year of radiology residency in Little Rock. Bennett is married to Laura Battle who is in her first year of dermatology residency. He is finishing his debut novel, *Failing*, which chronicles the personal and professional struggles of an aging pediatric heart surgeon.

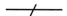

James S. Baumlin is distinguished Professor of English at Missouri State University in Springfield, Missouri, where he teaches Renaissance literature, the history of rhetoric, and creative nonfiction. He has authored and co-edited a dozen books and more than 100 essays, notes, and scholarly reviews.

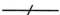

Brian Burton is an Arkansas native and third-generation graduate of University of Arkansas for Medical Sciences, following his grandfather (a general surgeon and Chief of Surgery of the US Army at Omaha Beach) and his father (a retired urologist). After obtaining a degree in microbiology from the University of Arkansas at Fayetteville, Brian worked as an orthotist, making braces for children with disabilities. During his third year of medical school, he shifted his sights away from orthopedic surgery and found his calling as an ObGyn. He joined The Woman's Clinic, P.A. in 2010 and has interests in minimally invasive gynecologic surgery including da Vinci Robotics, treatment of stress urinary incontinence, and high risk obstetrics including multiple gestations. Brian lives in Little Rock with his wife, three children, and a furry friend whose first choice of snack is not bananas. He is the first cousin of the editor.

Marcus Cafagña is the author of *The Broken World* (University of Illinois Press, 1996), a National Poetry Series selection, and Roman Fever (Invisible Cities Press, 2001). His poems and critical reviews have appeared in *The American Poetry Review, Ploughshares, Poets of the New Century, Poetry, Prairie Schooner*, and *The Southern Review*. He teaches poetry writing and coordinates the creative writing program at Missouri State University.

———/———

Shireen E. Campbell teaches courses in English and the first year Writing Program and directs the Writing Center at Davidson College. Her research, teaching, and publication interests range from writing center theory and practice to creative nonfiction, young adult fiction, and modern American and British literature. Her creative work has appeared in *Topograph: New Writing from the Carolinas and Beyond* (Novello Festival Press, 2010), *Double Lives, Reinvention, and Those We Leave Behind* (Wising Up Press, 2009), *Transformations: Reflections on Service* (Davidson College, 2009), and *Mom-Writers Literary Magazine*. She lives in Davidson, North Carolina, with her husband, two sons, one small dog, and one geriatric cat.

———/———

Gretchen A. Case is Assistant Professor in the Division of Medical Ethics and Humanities at the University of Utah School of Medicine. She received a BA in Speech Communication and History and an MA in Communication Studies from University of North Carolina–Chapel Hill, and a PhD in Performance Studies from University of California, Berkeley. Gretchen's interests lie in the many ways in which the arts and humanities intersect with medical arts and sciences. Her scholarly projects often combine communication, performance, disability theory, cultures of medicine, oral history, and ethnography. Gretchen has more than ten years of experience as a public historian, specializing in histories of science and medicine. She is currently developing empirically-based theatrical approaches to improving communication between health care providers and patients with Sydney Cheek-O'Donnell as part of their Initiative in Theatre, Performance, and Medicine. She lives in Salt Lake City with her husband and a four-year-old force of nature.

———/———

Jill Christman is an associate professor of English in Ball State University's Creative Writing Program and teaches creative nonfiction in Ashland University's low-residency MFA program (where she regularly presents at the River Teeth Nonfiction Conference). Her memoir, *Darkroom: A Family Exposure,* won the 2001 AWP Award Series in Creative Nonfiction and was reissued in 2011 by University of Georgia Press. Her first e-book, *Borrowed Babies: Apprenticing for Motherhood,* was released by Shebooks in September 2014. Recent nonfiction has appeared in *Brevity, Fourth Genre, River Teeth,* and many other journals, magazines, and anthologies. "Borrowed Babies," originally published in *Iron Horse Literary Review,* is listed as a notable essay in Best American Essays 2014. Jill lives in Muncie, Indiana with her husband, writer Mark Neely, and their two children. Visit her at http://www.jillchristman.com.

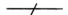

Chelsey Clammer received her MA in Women's Studies from Loyola University Chicago, and is currently enrolled in the Rainier Writing Workshop MFA program. She has been published in *The Rumpus, Essay Daily,* and *The Water~Stone Review* among many others. She is an award-winning essayist, and a freelance editor. Chelsey is the Managing Editor and Nonfiction Editor for *The Doctor T.J. Eckleburg Review,* as well as a columnist and workshop instructor for the journal. She is also the Nonfiction Editor for *Pithead Chapel* and Associate Essays Editor for *The Nervous Breakdown.* Her first collection of essays, *There Is Nothing Else to See Here,* is forthcoming from The Lit Pub, Winter 2014. Her second collection of essays, *BodyHome,* is forthcoming from Hopewell Publishing in Spring 2015. You can read more of her writing at www.chelseyclammer. com.

Jacqueline Conger ("Jackie") was born and raised in Arkansas. She completed a BA in chemistry at Arkansas State University in 2010, and graduated medical school from the University of Arkansas for Medical Sciences in 2014. She, her husband Matt (also a lifetime Arkansan), and their one-year old son, Charlie, have recently embarked on a new adventure in the Appalachian Mountains, where she is in her first year of ObGyn Residency at East Tennessee State University in Johnson City, Tennessee.

A pediatrician by training, **Sayantani Dasgupta** teaches in the Narrative Medicine Master's Program at Columbia University. She co-authored *Demon Slayers and Other Stories: Bengali Folk Tales* (Interlink, 1994), authored a memoir about her experience as a woman of color medical trainee, co-edited *Stories of Illness and Healing: Women Write their Bodies* (Kent State University Press, 2007), and co-edited *Globalization and Transnational Surrogacy in India: Outsourcing Life* (Lexington Books, 2014). She has published in *Ms.* (appearing on a 1992 cover with her mother), *Z. Magazine, JAMA, The Hasting's Center Report, The Lancet,* and *Literary Mama,* and is anthologized in many collections. She has written online for *Feministing.com, Racialicious.com, Adios, Barbie, From the Mixed Up Files of Middle-Grade Authors, The Feminist Wire, Sociological Images,* and *Everyday Feminism.* She is widely published in academia, and is often called on to give public talks in such forums as TEDxTalks. Learn more about her work at www.sayantanidasgupta.com.

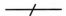

Kelli Dunham is the genderqueer nurse-comic-author-ex-nun hybrid so common in modern Brooklyn. Kelli was one of Velvet Park Magazine's 25 Significant Women of 2011 and was named to the 2012 Campus Pride Hotlist. She has appeared on Showtime and the Discovery Channel, nationwide at colleges, prides, and fundraisers, and even at the occasional livestock auction. Kelli is an RN and the author of five books of irreverent health-related nonfiction. Her fifth book, *Freak of Nurture* (Topside Press, 2013), is a collection of humorous essays and stories. The Lambda Literary Foundation website called Freak of Nurture "dynamic, generous, and smart . . . freakishly outstanding." Kelli has released four comedy CDs: "I am NOT a 12 Year Old Boy," "Almost Pretty," "Why Is the Fat One Always Angry," and "Trigger Warning," all of which are on regular rotation on Sirius/XM Satellite Radio's Rawdog Comedy Station and Pandora's Margaret Cho Station.

Lea Ervin holds an MA in Professional and Technical Writing from the University of Arkansas at Little Rock. She is a full-time instructor of English at Pulaski Technical College, where she teaches first year composition courses. Lea is an endometriosis awareness advocate, Smashing Pumpkins fan, yogi, writer, reader, Netflix junkie, live music enthusiast, tea drinker, friend, and daughter. Her academic interests include composition theory, rhetorical theory, and nonfiction writing— particularly the healing narrative. Her short nonfiction piece "Hold On" was featured on the April 22, 2014 broadcast of *Tales from the South*. Lea is a Helena, Arkansas, native and currently resides in Lonoke, Arkansas.

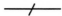

Jim Ferris is a poet and performance artist. He is author of *Slouching Towards Guantanamo* (Main Street Rag, 2011), *Facts of Life* (Parallel Press, 2005), and *The Hospital Poems*, which won the Main Street Rag Book Award in 2004. Ferris, who holds a doctorate in performance studies, has performed at the Kennedy Center, across the United States, and in Canada and Great Britain. Recent performance work includes the solo performance piece "Scars: A Love Story." Past president of the Society for Disability Studies, Jim has received awards for performance and mathematics as well as poetry and creative nonfiction. His writing has appeared in dozens of publications, ranging from *POETRY* to *Text & Performance Quarterly*, from the *Georgia Review* to weekly newspapers. He holds the Ability Center Endowed Chair in Disability Studies at the University of Toledo.

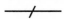

Lorrie Fredette creates site-specific investigations that examine beauty, harmony, and comfort to comprehend the incomprehensible of infection, pandemic, and plague. Lorrie holds a BFA in sculpture from the Herron School of Art/Indiana University. Her most recent solo shows were at Columbia Greene Community College in Hudson, New York, and the Garrison Art Center in Garrison, New York. A solo exhibition is scheduled for February 2015 at the Visual Arts Center of New Jersey. In 2014, she has been included in seven group shows. Publications include Faheem Haider's review of her installation at the Garrison Art Center in *Sculpture Magazine* (May 2014), and an interview with Megan Guerber in *SciArt in America* (April 2014). Cynthia-Reeves in New York represents her work.

Scott Huler has written on everything from the death penalty to bikini waxing, from NASCAR racing to the stealth bomber, for such newspapers as *The New York Times*, *The Washington Post*, the *Philadelphia Inquirer*, and the *Los Angeles Times* and such magazines as *Backpacker*, *Fortune*, and *ESPN*. His award-winning radio work has been heard on the public radio shows "All Things Considered," "Marketplace," and "Splendid Table." He was 2011 Piedmont Laureate and has served as a Knight-Wallace Fellow at Michigan in 2002-2003 and a Knight Science Journalism Fellow at MIT in 2014-2015. His work has appeared in numerous anthologies and collections, and he is at work on his seventh book of creative nonfiction, *A Delicious Country*, for which he is retracing the journey through the Carolinas in 1700-1701 of explorer John Lawson (www.lawsontrek.com). He lives in Raleigh, North Carolina, with his wife, the writer June Spence, and their two sons. Learn more about him at scotthuler.com.

————/————

Michelle Jarvis is a colon cancer survivor who has a permanent colostomy as a result of treatment. Through sharing her story, she hopes to help others with similar experiences. Michelle attended Catawba College in Salisbury, North Carolina, for undergraduate studies and Wake Forest University in Winston-Salem, North Carolina, for her graduate work. She lives in Thomasville, North Carolina, with her husband of 23 years, Ron, and four cats. She teaches English at Davidson County Community College in Lexington, North Carolina.

————/————

David Jay has been shooting fashion photography for the past twenty years. His work has been featured in *Vogue, Elle, Cosmopolitan, Style,* and *Shape,* and others. The focus of his photography shifted abruptly when a dear, young friend was diagnosed with breast cancer. Soon after, David began The SCAR Project, whose images have been published in the *The SCAR Project: Breast Cancer Is Not A Pink Ribbon* (The SCAR Project, 2011), *The New York Times, BBC, LIFE, Forbes, USA Today,* and countless other publications. *Bearing It All,* a documentary on the project, was released on the Style Network and won an Emmy Award. The SCAR Project is touring internationally. Another photographic series, *The Alabama Project: The Civil Rights of Health Care* is currently exhibited at the University of Alabama at Birmingham Cancer Center. David continues to illuminate oft unseen aspects of humanity with *The Unknown Soldier,* a series of large scale portraits of severely wounded young veterans returning home from the wars in Afghanistan and Iraq. David lives in New York.

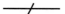

Douglas Kidd lives and works in Toledo, Ohio. Since his car accident, he achieved a BA in history and an MA in liberal studies with a concentration in disability studies. He is the founder/owner of Undistracted Driving Advocacy, LLC, works as a peer support specialist with Harbor (a mental health provider), and leads the Greater Toledo Brain Injury Support Group. Douglas serves as co-chair of the Accessibility/Transportation Committee of the Toledo/Lucas County Commission on Disabilities and is a member of the Board of Trustees of the Ability Center of Greater Toledo. He has published his poetry and academic writing in various publications, and has presented papers at the University of Toledo, The Ohio State University, and for The Society for Disability Studies.

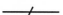

Heidi Kim is an assistant professor of English at the University of North Carolina at Chapel Hill. Her literary criticism on subjects such as William Faulkner, antislavery literature, and the Japanese American incarceration has appeared in journals including PMLA, the Walt Whitman Quarterly Review, and Philological Quarterly; her short stories have been published in Kartika Review and the Asian American Literary Review. This is her creative nonfiction debut.

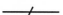

Philip Martin is the chief film and book critic, a columnist, and an editor for the *Arkansas Democrat-Gazette*. He is also the author the essay collections *The Shortstop's Son* (University of Arkansas Press, 1997) and *The Artificial Southerner* (University of Arkansas Press, 2001). His book of poetry, *The President Next Door: Poems, Songs and Journalism*, is forthcoming from Et Alia Press in spring 2015. The "monkey in the nose cone" at blood, dirt & angels (www.blooddirtangels.com), and co-producer of the ScreenPlay podcast, Philip has been a second baseman, rhythm guitarist, sportswriter, cop reporter, political columnist, and the executive editor of an alternative weekly. As a singer-songwriter, Philip appeared on the Merv Griffin Show in 1981, and has released the albums *Gastonia* (2013) and *Euclid Avenue* (2014). A finalist for the 2012 James Hearst Poetry Prize, he lives in Little Rock's Hillcrest neighborhood with his wife and editor, Karen, and three rescued terriers, Paris, Dublin, and Audi.

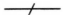

Stephen McNamee lost over seven years of his life to a severe physical illness (it was possibly closer to ten years depending on how much he's able to suppress at any given time). After healing through a combination of diet modification, acupuncture, supplements, meditation, and yoga, Stephen wrote, cast, produced, and starred in a sold-out sketch comedy show in New York City, *Casual Ambiguity*. He then wrote a young adult/urban fantasy novel, *It Would Like Suck to Die on a Tuesday: A Fairy Tale* (as yet unpublished). Stephen also mistakenly graduated from the University of Chicago Law School. In 2013, he wrote and filmed a short film, *Hold the Mayo* (currently making its way through the film festival circuit). In 2014, he created a web series, *There Are No Second Takes in Life . . . Take 2*. Every episode is between 15 seconds and 3 minutes and can be viewed at www.nosecondtakesinlife.com.

Jesse Nickles is an illustrator + graphic designer from Springfield, Missouri. He graduated from Missouri State University in 2010 with a BFA in graphic design. He works for Black Lantern Studios, a game developer, and has worked on many national and international games. He is co-owner of a print design service on Etsy called Atomica Press, which he runs with his lovely and talented wife Ashley.

Melissa Nicolas is an Associate Professor of English at the University of Nevada, Reno. Her most current work focuses on medical narratives and medical communication, particularly the patient/doctor interview. Her previous publications include work in *Inside Higher Education*, *The Chronicle of Higher Education*, *College Composition and Communication*, and the *Journal of College Writing*. Since originally writing this essay, she has had further abdominal surgery, creating even more scars on her stomach.

Kathryn Oliverio ("Kathy") is the academic editor and an adjunct professor at the University of Arkansas at Little Rock. She holds an MA in Professional and Technical Writing from the University of Arkansas at Little Rock. Her editorial work includes Berna Love's *Temple of Dreams: Taborian Hall and Its Dreamland Ballroom* (Lightning Source US Ltd, 2012) and Melissa Laney's *Forgotten but not Forgiven: Governor Ben T. Laney, Jr.* (as yet to be published).

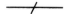

Chris Osmond is assistant professor of Leadership and Educational Studies at Appalachian State University in Boone, North Carolina. He earned his PhD in Culture, Curriculum, and Change from The University of North Carolina at Chapel Hill, his MA in Curriculum Studies and Teacher Education from Stanford University, and his BA in English and Spanish from Wesleyan University. His primary interest is in the preparation of caring professionals (e.g., teachers, doctors, nurses, social workers, allied health workers, counselors, clergy) for long, sustainable careers in the high-stress, low-resource environments that typifies those fields in our "measure-to-manage" era. His work adapts insights from the narrative medicine, aesthetic education, and expressive arts domains to work toward this goal. His other interests include curriculum theory and aesthetics, "reading together" as a professional formation site, and critical work on education policy as it defines the professional ambit of public school teachers. He is also a husband, a father, a drummer, and a runner.

Rianne Palazzolo was born and raised in North Little Rock and currently resides there. She has a passion for societal reform and has done a number of research projects about restorative justice. Her publications range in topics from government data reports regarding prison populations to Civil Rights and ACLU functionality for the *Criminal Justice Encyclopedia of Ethics*.

———/———

Jeffrey Paolano served in the U. S. Navy from 1964 to 1968 upon U.S.S. Cory DD-817 and in NCR-21, MCB-6 at Chu Lai. His works have been accepted for publication by *Frontier Tales*, *The Tanist's Wife Tales and other Stories* (alternative history), *Alive Day*, *Proud To Be: The Writings of American Warriors Vol. 3*, and *The Veteran's Writing Project*.

———/———

Samantha Plakun is a documentary film producer based in Brooklyn, New York. Regardless of form—whether through film, poetry or art—she loves storytelling. Sam believes that by telling our stories we learn who we are, and that by listening to the stories of others we become more compassionate. In 2012, she worked with incarcerated mothers at an alternative incarceration facility to create an exhibition of paper mache masks and poetry, entitled *Invisible Bodies*. *Written in Stitches* is Sam's first piece of published writing. Her favorite writer is Lydia Davis.

———/———

Andrea Razer is a veterinarian and mother to four cats, three boys, two dogs and one very bad squirrel. She grew up in Little Rock and graduated from Hendrix College in 2000. She attended the University of Missouri Veterinary School and joined Hillcrest Animal Hospital upon graduation. She is a life-long avid reader, and married her husband in a library. In her spare time she enjoys writing, photography, cutting out intricate paper snowflakes, and anything else that provides a creative outlet. If anyone knows how to re-seat the keys on an Apple laptop after they have been lifted off by a squirrel, they should contact Andrea without delay.

———/———

Heidi Andrea Restrepo Rhodes is a queer, Latina/second generation Colombian immigrant, poet/writer, scholar, photographer, and political activist. Both her scholarship and creative work focus on issues of social justice, historical memory, and collective healing, often with a nod to what is lost through various forms of violence, to the pain of absence, to the presence of ghosts, to what haunts us in the after. Her poetry has been seen or is forthcoming in places such as *As/Us Decolonial Love Issue, The Progressive, Mobius: A Journal for Social Change, Feminist Studies Journal, Raspa, Yellow Medicine Review, Descant, Write Bloody's* "We Will Be Shelter" and others. She currently lives in Brooklyn.

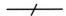

LaNita Rippere is a twenty-one-year breast cancer survivor who lives in Naples, Florida, and summers in Bar Harbor, Maine. She and her husband George, both retired from their jobs and thirty years in California, love the golfing and winter sun in Florida, and organic gardening and hiking the mountains of Acadia in the summer. Nita has a studio in Florida where she does facials and massage, and works part-time at Bella, a spa in Northeast Harbor, Maine. She believes you can maintain beauty and health at any age. She has helped reunite birth mothers with their adopted children, and also maintains her long-term sobriety by helping others find recovery from the disease of alcoholism.

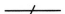

Aimee Ross is a nationally award-winning educator who's been teaching high school English at her alma mater in Loudonville, Ohio, for the past twenty-three years. Her passion for learning and teaching about the Holocaust has led to fellowships and study tours, published study guides and lessons (online and print), and numerous presentations, both nationally and internationally. Aimee is a contributing author to *Today I Made a Difference: A Collection of Inspirational Stories from America's Top Educators* (Adams Media, 2009), and she recently completed her MFA in Creative Non-Fiction Writing at Ashland University where she was taught by another writer in this volume, Jill Christman.

Maurice Carlos Ruffin is a graduate of the University of New Orleans Creative Writing Workshop, and a member of the Peauxdunque Writers Alliance and the Melanated Writers Collective. His work has appeared in *Redivider*, the *Apalachee Review*, and *Unfathomable City: A New Orleans Atlas* (University of California Press, 2013). He is the winner of the 2014 Iowa Review Fiction Award, the 2014 *So to Speak Journal* Short Story Award, and the 2014 William Faulkner Competition for *Novel in Progress*. He loves peanut butter and jelly; loud, but pretty music; and everything that Oscar Wilde ever said.

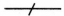

Emilie Staat's novel, *The Winter Circus*, is about an aerialist who grows up in the circus, runs away to New Orleans, and learns the value of falling. She is currently writing *Tango Face*, a memoir about what learning Argentine tango is teaching her about personhood, gender dynamics, and relationships.

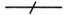

A childhood spent laboring on an archaeological dig in the Middle East honed **Jennifer Stager**'s interest in the stories we tell about material remains and prompted her to pursue a PhD in the history of art at University of California, Berkeley, which included fellowships from the Center for Advanced Study in the Visual Arts and the Getty Research Institute, as well as extensive travel. Each of her three children has five names and was born in a different city. Since returning home to the Bay Area in August 2013, Jennifer co-created the collaborative Unexpected Projects, which presents art in unusual spaces and ways. Jennifer is also revising for submission her book, *Puddles in the Morning*, or *The World Upside Down*, a coming-of-age account of losing her mother to early-onset Alzheimer's Disease and finding herself through that slow loss.

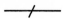

Annie Tucker is a writer, translator, and educator interested in the intersections of culture, disability, personal experience, and the arts. She received her PhD in Culture and Performance from UCLA in 2013 and is a lecturer for the Disability Studies minor there. Her translation of Indonesian author Eka Kurniawan's novel *Beauty is a Wound* is forthcoming from New Directions Books in 2015.

Clairese Webb received her BA in Writing and Biology from Drury University, and recently graduated medical school at the University of Arkansas for Medical Sciences. She is in her first year of anesthesiology residency in Oklahoma City. She enjoys writing nonfiction pieces about her experiences within and beyond the confines of hospital walls, and hopes her words may someday serve as a survival guide for prospective medical professionals.

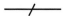

A media and entertainment professional, **Jason Wiest** has put his creative stamp on everything from newspapers to nightclubs. Formerly the Deputy Director of Communications for Gov. Mike Beebe, who was the nation's most popular Democratic governor while in office, Wiest is now a full-time entrepreneur. In addition to contract communications work, he runs Sway Nightclub, a downtown Little Rock establishment that opened in 2010. He also hosts *The Big Gay Radio Show* on the statewide community radio station KABF 88.3 FM. A Nebraska native, Wiest played the role of Herbie Husker, the mascot for the University of Nebraska-Lincoln, where he earned his Bachelor's of Journalism degree as well as the title of Capital One's "National Mascot of the Year." In 2010, he completed his MBA at the University of Arkansas at Little Rock. His volunteer work includes service on the Board of Directors for Ballet Arkansas, the state's only professional dance company, as well as the for the Stonewall Democratic Caucus of Arkansas.

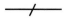

Andrea Zekis is a cartographer, amateur stilt walker, and advocate to Arkansas's transgender population. She has called Little Rock home since 2005. In 2014, she co-founded the Arkansas Transgender Equality Coalition (ArTEC) as a non-profit statewide transgender organization focused on advancing education, resources, and inclusive communities in the Natural State. Andrea also serves as a consultant to the Human Rights Campaign's Project One America. For her advocacy, *Arkansas Times* honored Andrea as an Arkansas visionary in 2014. She previously spent five years as a local television news producer, and currently works in the mapping offices of the Arkansas Highway and Transportation Department. Andrea is a native of Munster, Indiana and is a graduate of both the University of Evansville and Syracuse University. She loves dogs, music, travel, the outdoors, watching baseball and hockey, making people laugh, and living authentically.

CPSIA information can be obtained
at www.ICGtesting.com
Printed in the USA
FFOW02n2153011215
19156FF